GAO

Report to the Committee on Finance, U.S. Senate

I0426306

July 2012

MEDICAID

States Reported Billions More in Supplemental Payments in Recent Years

To access this report electronically, scan this QR Code.

Don't have a QR code reader? Several are available for free online.

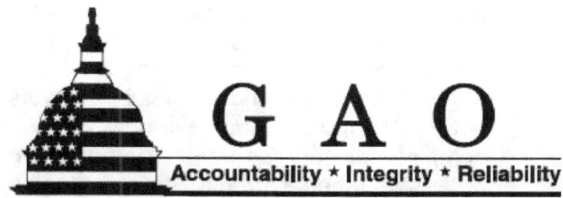

GAO

Accountability ★ Integrity ★ Reliability

GAO-12-694

MEDICAID

States Reported Billions More in Supplemental Payments in Recent Years

Highlights of GAO-12-694, a report to the Committee on Finance, U.S. Senate

Why GAO Did This Study

GAO designated Medicaid a high-risk program because of concerns about its size, growth, and inadequate fiscal oversight. The program cost the federal government and states an estimated $383 billion in fiscal year 2010. In addition to regular Medicaid payments to providers, states make supplemental payments, including DSH payments, which are intended to offset the uncompensated costs of care provided to uninsured individuals and Medicaid beneficiaries. States also make other supplemental payments, which we refer to as non-DSH supplemental payments, to hospitals and other providers, for example, to help offset the costs of care provided to Medicaid beneficiaries. GAO and others have raised concerns about the transparency of states' Medicaid supplemental payments. GAO was asked to provide information on supplemental payments.

GAO examined (1) how much states reported paying in supplemental Medicaid payments during fiscal year 2010 and (2) how non-DSH supplemental payments reported during 2010 compared with those reported during 2006 and reasons for differences. GAO analyzed CMS's Medicaid expenditure data for all states and information from CMS and other sources about non-DSH supplemental payments in a nongeneralizable sample of 11 states selected to capture a mix of relevant characteristics.

In its comments on a draft of GAO's report, HHS stated that HHS and CMS will continue their ongoing efforts to improve states' reporting of supplemental Medicaid payments.

View GAO-12-694. For more information, contact Katherine Iritani at (202) 512-7114 or iritan k@gao.gov.

What GAO Found

States reported $32 billion in Medicaid supplemental payments during fiscal year 2010, but the exact amount of supplemental payments is unknown because state reporting was incomplete. On expenditure reports used to obtain federal funds filed with the Department of Health and Human Services' (HHS) Centers for Medicare & Medicaid Services (CMS), states reported the following:

- A total of $17.6 billion in Disproportionate Share Hospital (DSH) payments. The 10 states reporting the largest total DSH payments in fiscal year 2010 accounted for more than 70 percent of the nationwide total, with 4 states—New York, California, Texas, and New Jersey—accounting for almost half (47 percent). DSH payments as a percentage of total Medicaid payments varied considerably—ranging from 1 to 17 percent—among the 50 states that reported DSH payments.

- A total of $14.4 billion in non-DSH supplemental payments to hospitals and other providers. Because not all states reported these payments separately, complete information is not available. Like DSH payments, non-DSH supplemental payments as a percentage of total state Medicaid spending varied considerably—also ranging from 1 to 17 percent—among the 30 reporting states. These payments can also constitute a large portion of states' expenditures for particular categories of services, such as inpatient or outpatient hospital, nursing facility, or physician and surgical services. For example, non-DSH supplemental payments for inpatient hospital services ranged from 1 to 48 percent of state expenditures for these services among reporting states.

CMS officials told GAO that they were taking steps to improve states' reporting of non-DSH supplemental payments, including working with states to train staff on reporting of payments and on identifying and resolving reporting problems.

States' reported non-DSH supplemental payments were more than $8 billion higher during 2010 than during 2006, the year for which GAO previously reported on the amount of these payments. More complete state reporting of payments and new and modified supplemental payments were factors in this increase. The information available to identify changes from 2006 to 2010 came from 39 states that separately reported non-DSH supplemental payments during either 2006 or 2010 or both. Most of the increase was from the 15 states that reported some payments in both years and reported higher non-DSH supplemental payments during 2010 than 2006. In addition, most of the reported increase was for inpatient hospital services. In 11 selected states, GAO found that new and modified supplemental payments contributed to some increases. For example, new and modified supplemental payments for hospital services in Colorado and Illinois are estimated to increase the states' non-DSH supplemental payments by about $300 million and $1 billion per year, respectively. However, data limitations prevented GAO from quantifying the full extent to which the increase was attributable to new and modified payments. In light of the apparent increase in non-DSH supplemental payments, ongoing federal efforts to improve the completeness of reporting are important for effective oversight and to better understand the payments' role in financing Medicaid services.

_____ United States Government Accountability Office

Contents

Figures

Abbreviations

CMS   Centers for Medicare & Medicaid Services
DSH   Disproportionate Share Hospital
FMR   Financial Management Report
HHS   Department of Health and Human Services
UPL   Upper Payment Limit

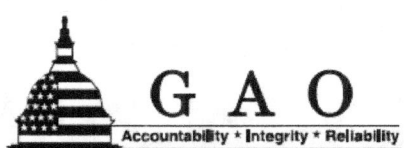
July 20, 2012

The Honorable Max Baucus
Chairman
The Honorable Orrin G. Hatch
Ranking Member
Committee on Finance
United States Senate

In 2003, GAO designated Medicaid—the federal-state program that finances health care for certain low-income individuals—as a high-risk program because of growing concern about its size, growth, and inadequate fiscal oversight, including federal oversight of supplemental payments.[1] Supplemental payments are separate from and in addition to payments made at a state's regular Medicaid rates. The federal government and states share in the cost of Medicaid, which in fiscal year 2010 totaled about $383 billion.[2] As the program continues to grow in cost and significance, policymakers and others need better information to manage the program, including information about the amount and purposes of Medicaid provider payments. GAO has found that this includes a need for information about supplemental payments, which have contributed to Medicaid cost growth in the past.[3]

Medicaid financing is a joint responsibility of the federal government and states. States pay qualified health care providers for covered services provided to Medicaid beneficiaries, and then seek reimbursement for the federal share of those payments. Under the Social Security Act, state Medicaid payments are required to be consistent with efficiency, economy, and quality of care and sufficient to enlist an adequate number

---

[1]GAO, *High-Risk Series: An Update*, GAO-11-278 (Washington, D.C.: February 2011).

[2]This figure represents combined federal and state Medicaid expenditures for provider services in fiscal year 2010, the latest year for which data were available when we conducted our work. For the purpose of this report, expenditures for administration are not included. Medicaid programs are administered by the 50 states, the District of Columbia, Puerto Rico, and four U.S. territories—American Samoa, Guam, the Northern Mariana Islands, and the U.S. Virgin Islands.

[3]See, for example, GAO, *Medicaid: CMS Needs More Information on the Billions of Dollars Spent on Supplemental Payments*, GAO-08-614 (Washington, D.C.: May 30, 2008).

of providers. The federal government oversees states' Medicaid programs and, by a formula established in law, pays from half to more than three-fourths of each state's allowable Medicaid expenditures.[4]

In addition to their regular Medicaid payments, all states make supplemental payments that are also matched by federal funds.[5] For the purposes of this report, we classified supplemental payments into two general categories: Disproportionate Share Hospital (DSH) and non-DSH supplemental payments.

- **DSH payments** are payments to hospitals that serve a disproportionate share of low-income and Medicaid patients to help offset hospitals' uncompensated costs for serving these individuals.[6] DSH payments are required by law and are limited (or capped) at the facility-specific level and the state level.

- **Non-DSH supplemental payments** are other supplemental payments that states have made under Medicaid Upper Payment Limit (UPL) regulations. The UPL is the ceiling on federal matching funds for Medicaid payments and is based on an estimate of what Medicare would pay for comparable services.[7] Because states' regular Medicaid payments are often less than the UPL, most states have established supplemental payments above regular Medicaid rates, but within the UPL. Unlike regular Medicaid payments, which are paid on the basis of covered Medicaid services provided to

---

[4]Under a statutory formula, the federal government may reimburse from 50 to 83 percent of a state's Medicaid expenditures for services. States with lower per capita incomes receive higher federal matching rates. 42 U.S.C. §§ 1396b(a), 1396d(b).

[5]In this report, we use the term state to refer to the 50 states and the District of Columbia. We do not include Puerto Rico or the U.S. territories of American Samoa, Guam, the Northern Mariana Islands, or the U.S. Virgin Islands (which have Medicaid programs) because they did not report supplemental Medicaid payments in 2010.

[6]See 42 U.S.C. §§ 1396a(13)(A)(iv), 1396r-4.

[7]Medicare is the federal health program that covers seniors aged 65 and older and some disabled persons. Separate UPLs exist for inpatient services provided by hospitals, nursing facilities, and intermediate care facilities for individuals with intellectual disabilities, and for outpatient services provided by hospitals and clinics. These UPLs are applied on an aggregate basis to three categories of providers: local (nonstate) government-owned or government-operated facilities, state-government-owned or state-government-operated facilities, and privately owned and operated facilities. See 42 C.F.R. §§ 447.272, 447.321 (2011).

Medicaid beneficiaries through an automated claims process, these non-DSH supplemental payments are not necessarily made on the basis of claims submitted for the delivery of specific services to particular patients. States have made non-DSH payments to hospitals, nursing homes, physician groups, and other Medicaid providers.[8] Unlike DSH payments, states are not required to make non-DSH supplemental payments, and payments are not subject to overall state spending or provider-specific limits.

For more than a decade, we and others have reported concerns with the oversight and transparency of states' financing arrangements involving supplemental payments.[9] Our past work had found that the Centers for Medicare & Medicaid Services (CMS)—the agency within the Department of Health and Human Services (HHS) with oversight responsibility for Medicaid—lacked information on the billions of dollars spent on supplemental payments, including the magnitude of payments, how individual states were calculating payment amounts, the providers that received the payments, and the purposes for which they were received. States have flexibility for making such payments, which could greatly affect the total Medicaid payments that individual providers receive. To the extent that some providers receive a substantial proportion of their Medicaid payments as supplemental payments that are not directly linked to services or costs, it becomes difficult to compare payment levels across providers or to evaluate the impact of Medicaid payment policies.

In May 2008, we reported that for federal fiscal year 2006, states reported making at least $23 billion in supplemental payments, with a federal share totaling over $13 billion. States reported $17 billion in DSH payments and $6 billion in non-DSH supplemental payments. However, the exact amount of non-DSH supplemental payments was unknown because states did not report all of their payments to CMS separately from payments based on their regular payment rates.[10] In the absence of transparent information about how much states are spending on non-DSH supplemental payments, the relative significance of non-DSH supplemental payments in comparison to regular Medicaid payments or

---

[8]In this report, we use the terms non-DSH payments and non-DSH supplemental payments interchangeably.

[9]A list of related GAO products can be found at the end of this report.

[10]GAO-08-614.

DSH payments has not been clear. Beginning in fiscal year 2010, CMS implemented new expenditure reporting procedures under which states were to report certain non-DSH supplemental payments separately from their regular payments.

Given the lack of transparency of states' supplemental Medicaid payments, members of Congress and others have expressed interest in them. You asked for information regarding how much states reported spending on supplemental payments, including changes in reported payments since 2006, the year for which GAO had previously reported on these payments, and oversight of supplemental payments.[11] This report addresses the following questions:

1. How much did states report paying in supplemental Medicaid payments during fiscal year 2010?

2. How did non-DSH supplemental payments reported during 2010 compare with those payments reported during 2006, and what were reasons for differences?

To determine how much states reported paying for supplemental Medicaid payments during 2010, we analyzed Medicaid expenditure data that CMS had finalized for federal fiscal year 2010.[12] These are data that states reported to CMS during fiscal year 2010 using a standardized form, the CMS-64, to claim federal matching funds.[13] To understand Medicaid supplemental payments and processes for reporting these payments, we reviewed relevant federal laws, regulations, and guidance and

---

[11] In a separate report, we plan to examine information available for overseeing DSH and non-DSH supplemental payments.

[12] Throughout this report, the term fiscal year refers to the federal fiscal year.

[13] We include payments reported on the CMS-64s submitted for the four quarters of fiscal year 2010. States are to file their expenditure reports within 30 days of the end of a quarter. CMS reviews this information and, if necessary, obtains clarifications or revisions before finalizing the data. States may make adjustments to their expenditure reports for up to 2 years. Adjustments are made to the payment amounts reported during the fiscal year in which a state reports an adjustment rather than the fiscal year in which the original payment was made. For example, if a state reported in fiscal year 2010 that it made an overpayment in fiscal year 2009, the adjustment would be treated as a reduction to the amount the state reported paying during fiscal year 2010. We did not include any adjustments to payments reported during fiscal year 2010 that may have been included in quarterly CMS-64s submitted after fiscal year 2010.

interviewed CMS officials. We examined the amount of DSH and non-DSH supplemental payments reported by individual states and the nationwide totals, and we analyzed the amounts reported for different categories of service. In addition, to better understand the contribution of supplemental payments to state Medicaid spending, we examined the share of state spending attributed to supplemental payments.

To determine how non-DSH supplemental payments reported during 2010 compared with those payments reported during 2006, we analyzed 2006 and 2010 expenditures for non-DSH supplemental payments that states reported to CMS separately from their other payments.[14] To examine reasons for differences between 2006 and 2010 in reported non-DSH supplemental payments, and to obtain additional information about states' reports of these payments, we obtained information from CMS and public sources about non-DSH supplemental payments in a judgmental sample of 11 states selected to include a mix of relevant characteristics. Our selections included some states that separately reported such payments in only 1 of the 2 years, and states that differed in absolute and relative changes in reported non-DSH supplemental payments and changes in categories of payment. The information we used to select states included published information, as well as preliminary information from CMS.[15] For each of these states, we examined information that could help explain net changes from 2006 to 2010 in the state's reported non-DSH supplemental payment amounts, such as establishment of new non-DSH supplemental payments, modification of existing non-DSH supplemental payments, or a change in reporting that would result in an increase or decrease in the state's reported payments. The information we reviewed included information that states submitted to CMS prior to changing their supplemental payments.[16] When this information indicated that a supplemental payment had been established, modified, or terminated, we examined documentation of how much the state's payments were expected to

---

[14]We obtained data about expenditures reported during fiscal year 2006 as part of work we reported in 2008. See GAO-08-614.

[15]We selected Arkansas, Colorado, Georgia, Illinois, Maine, Massachusetts, Missouri, North Carolina, Pennsylvania, South Carolina, and Texas. Expenditure data from fiscal year 2010 had not been finalized at the time we made our selections.

[16]To receive federal matching funds, states must obtain approval from CMS for any changes to their Medicaid payment rates.

change as a result. Information from these states cannot be generalized to other states. A more detailed description of our scope and methodology can be found in appendix I.

To assess the reliability of the data on supplemental Medicaid payments reported to CMS by the states in 2006 and 2010, we reviewed the procedures CMS used to obtain and compile the data and discussed the data with CMS officials. We determined that the data were sufficiently reliable to describe the amounts of supplemental payments that were reported separately by states during 2006 and 2010. Because some states did not separately report all of their non-DSH supplemental payments during 2006 or 2010, our analysis only captures changes in non-DSH supplemental payments that were separately reported. Information is not available that would have allowed us to quantify the extent to which states did not separately report these supplemental payments. Therefore, we may not be capturing the full amount of states' supplemental payments or the degree to which they have changed over time. We did not examine whether changes in non-DSH supplemental payments were associated with changes in states' regular Medicaid payments.

We conducted this performance audit from November 2011 to July 2012 in accordance with generally accepted government auditing standards. Those standards require that we plan and perform the audit to obtain sufficient, appropriate evidence to provide a reasonable basis for our findings and conclusions based on our audit objectives. We believe that the evidence obtained provides a reasonable basis for our findings and conclusions based on our audit objectives.

Background

Title XIX of the Social Security Act established Medicaid as a federal-state partnership that finances health care for low-income individuals, including children, families, the aged, and the disabled.[17] Medicaid is an open-ended entitlement program and provided health coverage for an estimated 53.9 million individuals in 2010.[18] Within broad federal requirements, each state administers and operates its Medicaid

---

[17] 42 U.S.C. § 1396a et seq. (2010).

[18] See Department of Health and Human Services, *2011 Actuarial Report on the Financial Outlook for Medicaid* (Washington, D.C.: 2012).

program in accordance with a state Medicaid plan, which must be approved by CMS. A state Medicaid plan details the populations that are served, the categories of services that are covered (such as inpatient hospital services, nursing facility services, and physician services), and the methods for calculating payments to providers. The state Medicaid plan also describes the supplemental payments established by the state and specifies which providers are eligible to receive supplemental payments and what categories of service are covered. Any changes a state wishes to make in its Medicaid plan, such as establishing new payments or changing methods for developing provider payment rates, must be submitted to CMS for review and approval as a state plan amendment. States may also receive approval from CMS for a waiver from certain Medicaid requirements in order to conduct a Medicaid demonstration, and these demonstrations may include supplemental payments. These demonstrations allow states to test new approaches to deliver or pay for health services through Medicaid. Under certain demonstrations, a state may cover populations or services that would not otherwise be eligible for federal Medicaid funding under federal rules. Some states, including California and Massachusetts, have also in recent years been allowed to make supplemental payments under Medicaid demonstrations. The terms and conditions governing such demonstrations are specific to each demonstration.

All states make supplemental Medicaid payments to certain providers. DSH payments are made to hospitals and cannot exceed the unreimbursed cost of furnishing inpatient and outpatient services to Medicaid beneficiaries and the uninsured.[19] Non-DSH supplemental

---

[19]Under the Patient Protection and Affordable Care Act, the annual cap on the amount of federal matching funds available for DSH payments nationwide will be reduced in fiscal years 2014 through 2020. See Pub. L. No. 111-148, §§ 2551, 10201(e)(1)(B), 10201(f), 124 Stat. 119, 312, 920, 922 (Mar. 23, 2010), as amended by Pub. L. No. 111-152, § 1203(b), 124 Stat. 1029, 1053 (Mar. 30, 2010). Annual reductions in federal DSH funding during these years range from $500 million to $5.6 billion, and reductions for all years total $18.1 billion. The Middle Class Tax Relief and Job Creation Act of 2012 extended these reductions through fiscal year 2021. See Pub. L. No. 112-96, § 3203, 126 Stat. 156, 193 (Feb. 22, 2012). States' DSH allotments—the maximum amount of federal matching funds that each state may receive for DSH payments—were first established in 1991 based on each state's historical DSH spending. See the Medicaid Voluntary Contribution and Provider-Specific Tax Amendments of 1991, Pub. L. No. 102-234, § 3, 105 Stat. 1793, 1799-1804 (Dec. 12, 1991) (codified, as amended, at 42 U.S.C. § 1396r-4(f)). Congress has amended requirements for calculating these DSH allotments since their establishment. Currently, CMS calculates each state's fiscal year DSH allotment using a statutorily defined formula.

payments can be made to hospitals or other providers (such as nursing homes or groups of physicians) for any category of service provided on a fee-for-service basis.[20] For example, a state might make non-DSH supplemental payments on a quarterly basis to county-owned nursing facilities that serve low-income populations to fill the gap between what regular Medicaid rates pay toward the cost of services and higher payments permitted through the UPL. Supplemental payments are typically made for services provided on a fee-for-service basis, rather than those provided through Medicaid managed care contracts.[21] Non-DSH supplemental payments need to be approved by CMS.

To obtain the federal matching funds for Medicaid payments made to providers, each state files a quarterly expenditure report to CMS—the CMS-64. This form compiles state payments in over 20 categories of medical services, such as inpatient hospital services and outpatient hospital services. States are required to report total DSH payments made to hospitals and mental health facilities separately from other Medicaid payments in order to receive reimbursement for them. From 2001 through 2009, when completing the CMS-64 to obtain federal matching funds for non-DSH supplemental payments, states combined their non-DSH supplemental payments with their regular payments—those made using states' regular Medicaid payment rates. During this period, CMS requested that states report their non-DSH supplemental payments in a separate informational section of the CMS-64 that was not the basis for states receipt of federal matching funds. Instead, states received federal matching funds based on their reports of expenditure totals that included both regular and non-DSH supplemental payments. In 2008, we found that states reported making $6.3 billion in non-DSH supplemental payments during fiscal year 2006, but that not all states reported their non-DSH supplemental payments separately from other expenditures of the same type.[22] Starting with the first quarter of fiscal year 2010, CMS's new reporting procedures requested that states report certain non-DSH

[20]Including regular and supplemental payments, states reported spending about $284 billion for fee-for-service benefits during fiscal year 2010, representing about 73 percent of Medicaid spending for benefits during that year.

[21]Federal law generally prohibits states from making separate payment for services covered under a managed care contract. See 42 C.F.R. § 438.60 (2011).

[22]See GAO-08-614. At the time of our review, fiscal year 2006 was the most recent year for which data were available.

supplemental payments separately from their regular payments on the section of the CMS-64 used to claim federal matching funds.[23] However, CMS continues to provide federal matching funds to states that report these payments in combination with regular payments on this form.

States Reported $32 Billion in Supplemental Medicaid Payments during Fiscal Year 2010, but the Exact Amount of Supplemental Payments Is Unknown

The data CMS finalized for fiscal year 2010 show that states and the federal government spent at least $32 billion for DSH and non-DSH supplemental payments during fiscal year 2010, with the federal share of these payments totaling at least $19.8 billion. States reported $17.6 billion in DSH payments and $14.4 billion in non-DSH supplemental payments during fiscal year 2010, but state reporting of non-DSH supplemental payments separately from regular payments was incomplete, so the exact amount of non-DSH supplemental payments is unknown.

States Reported $17.6 Billion in DSH Payments during Fiscal Year 2010

States reported $17.6 billion in DSH payments during fiscal year 2010, with the federal government reimbursing states $9.9 billion for its share of these payments. Fifty of the 51 states reported making DSH payments during fiscal year 2010, with total reported payments ranging from about $650,000 for South Dakota to over $3.1 billion for New York.[24] The 10 states reporting the largest total DSH payments in fiscal year 2010

---

[23]Separate reporting applies to six categories of service: inpatient hospital services, outpatient hospital services, nursing facility services, physician and surgical services, other practitioners' services, and intermediate care facility services. CMS did not request that states report non-DSH supplemental payments for all categories of services separately from their regular payments. For example, CMS did not request separate reporting of non-DSH supplemental payments for mental health services or home health services. The section of the CMS-64 that states were requested to use to report non-DSH supplemental payments during fiscal year 2006 allowed reporting of such payments for all categories of service for which the state could report regular payments.

[24]Massachusetts did not report DSH payments in fiscal year 2010 because it conducted a Medicaid demonstration that exempted it from making DSH payments. This demonstration, called the MassHealth Medicaid demonstration, was approved by CMS in 2005 and has been approved through June 30, 2014.

accounted for more than 70 percent of the $17.6 billion nationwide total, and the 4 states with the largest total DSH payments—New York, California, Texas, and New Jersey—accounted for almost half (47 percent) of the nationwide total.

In assessing the contribution of DSH payments to each state's overall spending, we found that DSH payments as a percentage of states' reported Medicaid payments varied considerably among the states.[25] Among states that reported DSH payments, the percentage ranged from less than 1 percent (Arizona, Delaware, North Dakota, South Dakota, Wisconsin, and Wyoming) to 17 percent (New Hampshire). Figure 1 provides information on the amount of each state's DSH payments and each state's DSH payments as a percentage of its total Medicaid expenditures. (App. II lists each state's reported DSH payments during fiscal year 2010, the federal share of those payments, the state's total Medicaid payments, and each state's total reported DSH payment as a percentage of the state's total Medicaid payments and of total nationwide DSH payments.)

---

[25]We use the term Medicaid payments to refer to a state's medical assistance payments, which are the total Medicaid payments made by a state for medical services, including supplemental payments, but not including administrative costs.

Figure 1: DSH Payments Reported by States during Federal Fiscal Year 2010, in Dollars and as a Percentage of the State's Total Medicaid Payments

Dollars | **Percentages**

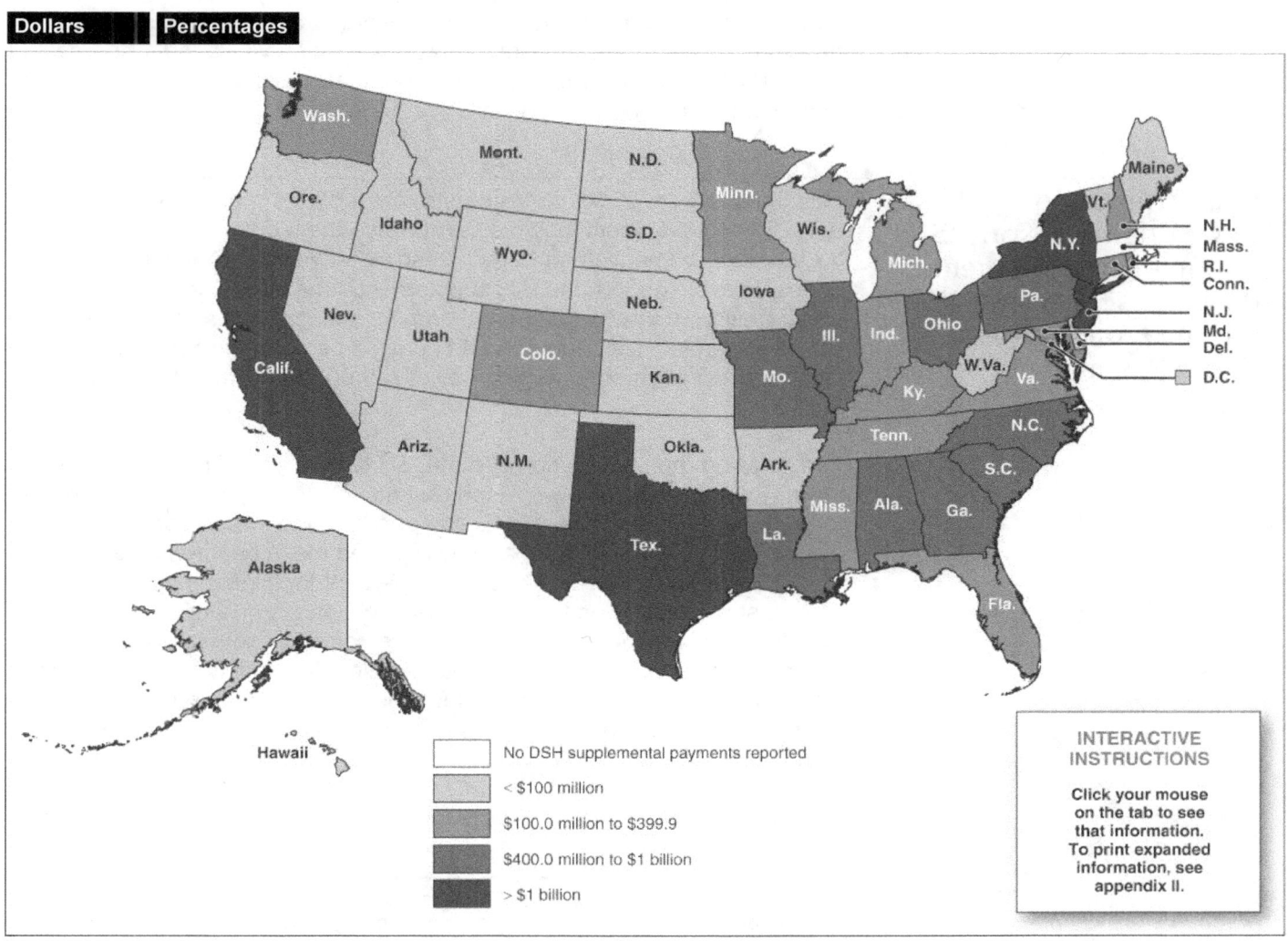

Legend:
- No DSH supplemental payments reported
- < $100 million
- $100.0 million to $399.9
- $400.0 million to $1 billion
- > $1 billion

INTERACTIVE INSTRUCTIONS

Click your mouse on the tab to see that information. To print expanded information, see appendix II.

Sources: GAO analysis of CMS files (data); Map Resources (map).

Notes: Puerto Rico and the U.S. territories that operate Medicaid programs are not included on this map because they were not authorized to make DSH payments in fiscal year 2010. Massachusetts did not report DSH payments in fiscal year 2010 because it conducted a Medicaid demonstration that exempted it from making DSH payments. This demonstration, called the MassHealth Medicaid demonstration, was approved by CMS in 2005 and has been approved through June 30, 2014.

The majority of DSH payments were to hospitals for traditional inpatient and outpatient services. During fiscal year 2010, 83 percent of the nationwide total of reported DSH payments ($14.7 billion) was paid to hospitals for traditional inpatient and outpatient services and 17 percent of the total ($2.9 billion) was paid to mental health facilities for inpatient and outpatient mental health services.[26]

States Reported $14.4 Billion in Non-DSH Supplemental Payments during Fiscal Year 2010, but the Exact Amount of These Payments Is Not Known

During fiscal year 2010, states separately reported making $14.4 billion in non-DSH supplemental payments (of which the federal share was $9.9 billion), primarily for inpatient hospital services.[27] Beginning in 2010, states were to report non-DSH supplemental payments on the CMS-64 separately from their regular payments for six categories of service. Thirty states separately reported non-DSH payments during fiscal year 2010, with reported payments ranging from $125,000 for Vermont to $3.1 billion for Texas.

In assessing the contribution of non-DSH supplemental payments to each state's overall spending, we found that non-DSH supplemental payments as a percentage of states' Medicaid spending also varied considerably across the 30 states that separately reported these payments, ranging from 1 percent for Vermont to over 17 percent for Illinois. Figure 2 provides information on the amount of each state's non-DSH supplemental payments and each state's non-DSH supplemental payments as a percentage of its total Medicaid expenditures. (App. II lists each state's reported non-DSH supplemental payments during fiscal year 2010, the federal share of those payments, the state's total Medicaid

[26]Traditional inpatient and outpatient services include services that are furnished in a hospital for the care and treatment of inpatients and outpatients, other than services provided in mental health facilities. See 42 C.F.R. §§ 440.10, 440.20 (2011).

[27]The federal share was larger for non-DSH supplemental payments ($9.9 billion of $14.4 billion) than for DSH payments ($9.9 billion of $17.6 billion) because states could claim an enhanced matching rate for non-DSH supplemental payments under the American Recovery and Reinvestment Act of 2009, but were explicitly prohibited from claiming an enhanced match for DSH payments. Under the American Recovery and Reinvestment Act of 2009, as amended by Public Law 111-226, states could claim an enhanced matching rate for non-DSH supplemental payments from October 1, 2008, through June 30, 2011. Pub. L. No. 111-226, § 201, 124 Stat. 2389, 2393 (Aug. 10, 2010), amending Pub. L. No. 111-5, § 5001, 123 Stat. 115, 496 (Feb. 17, 2009).

payments, and each state's total reported non-DSH supplemental payments as a percentage of the state's total Medicaid payments and of total nationwide non-DSH supplemental payments.)

Figure 2: Non-DSH Supplemental Payments Separately Reported by States during Federal Fiscal Year 2010, in Dollars and as a Percentage of the State's Total Medicaid Payments

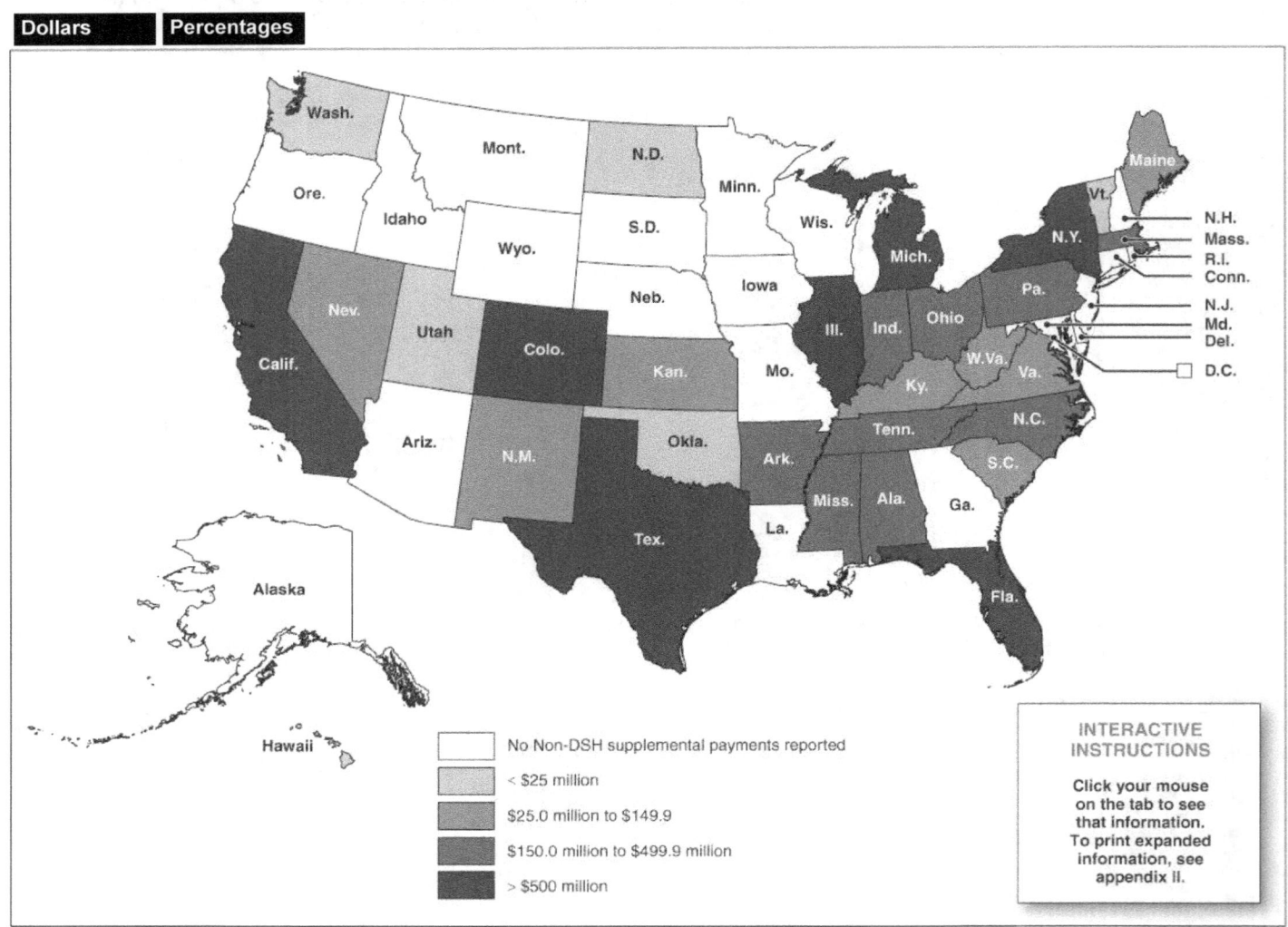

Sources: GAO analysis of CMS files (data); Map Resources (map).

Note: Puerto Rico and the U.S. territories that operate Medicaid programs are not included on this map because they did not report any supplemental Medicaid payments during 2010.

Of the six categories of service for which states reported making non-DSH supplemental payments, states reported the largest amount of payments for inpatient hospital services. States reported $11 billion in non-DSH supplemental payments for inpatient services (with a federal share of $7.7 billion). States reported $1.8 billion in non-DSH supplemental payments for outpatient services (with a federal share of $1.15 billion). (See fig. 3.)

Figure 3: Non-DSH Supplemental Payments Separately Reported during 2010 by Category of Service (Dollars in Millions)

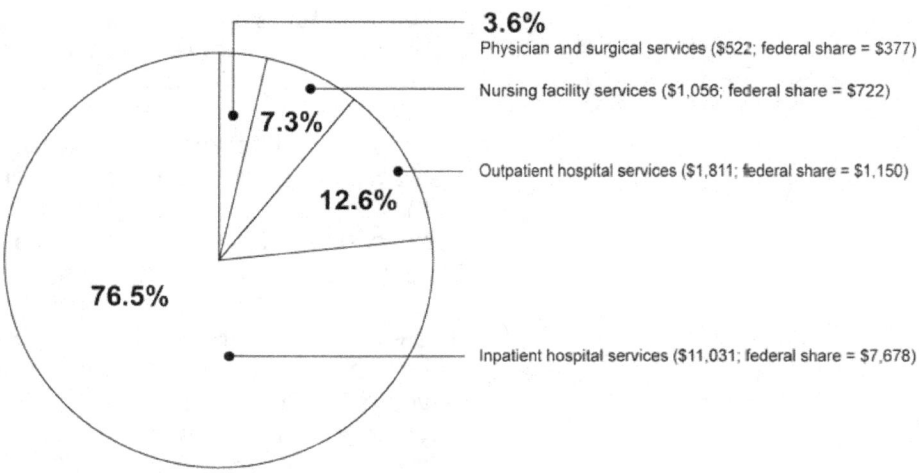

Source: GAO analysis of CMS-64 expenditure data.

Note: Combined non-DSH supplemental payments for other practitioners' services and for intermediate care facility services totaled less than 0.01 percent of states' total Medicaid payments reported during fiscal year 2010.

The proportion of a state's reported expenditures that were non-DSH supplemental payments varied across states and categories of service. In some states, non-DSH supplemental payments represented very little of the state's reported expenditures for a category of service, while in other states, non-DSH supplemental payments represented more than one-third of the state's reported expenditures for a category of service. For example,

- 27 states separately reported non-DSH supplemental payments for inpatient hospital services, and the percentage of their expenditures for inpatient hospital services that were non-DSH supplemental payments ranged from less than 1 percent (Virginia and Washington) to 48 percent (Tennessee);[28]

- 13 states separately reported non-DSH supplemental payments for outpatient hospital services, and the percentage of their expenditures for outpatient hospital services that were non-DSH supplemental payments ranged from less than 1 percent (Texas) to 57 percent (Illinois); and

- 16 states separately reported non-DSH supplemental payments for physician and surgical services, and the percentage of their expenditures for physician and surgical hospital services that were non-DSH supplemental payments ranged from less than 1 percent (Oklahoma) to 34 percent (West Virginia).

See appendix II for more information about each state's reported total and non-DSH supplemental payments for inpatient hospital services, outpatient hospital services, nursing facility services, physician and surgical services, other practitioners' services, and intermediate care facility services.

The exact amount of non-DSH supplemental payments nationwide is unknown, in part because not all states that made non-DSH supplemental payments in 2010 reported them on the CMS-64 separately from regular payments, and some states separately reported some but not all of their non-DSH supplemental payments. For example, Georgia reported $0 for non-DSH supplemental payments during fiscal year 2010, but according to CMS, it made non-DSH supplemental payments of $120.6 million for nursing home services during 2010.

CMS officials told us that they are aware that some states did not separately report all of their non-DSH supplemental payments. Officials stated that they have taken, and are taking, steps to improve states' reporting of non-DSH supplemental payments for the six categories of service. They told us that after revising the form CMS-64 to include lines for separate reporting of certain non-DSH supplemental payments, they monitored states' reports of these payments and, as a result, they learned

---

[28]Total expenditures for inpatient hospital services for this analysis consisted of regular Medicaid payments, DSH supplemental payments, non-DSH supplemental payments, and payments to help support graduate medical education.

that some states had not reported these payments separately. They then took steps to improve states' reporting of these payments, for example, by training state staff in the use of the revised form CMS-64 and asking regional CMS staff to work with states to identify and resolve reporting problems. CMS officials also noted, however, that some states encountered technical difficulties with their state databases. For example, CMS officials told us that the data systems used by some states in 2010 did not permit them to separate the non-DSH supplemental payments from their regular payments. CMS officials confirmed that states did not separately report all non-DSH supplemental payments in 2010 and acknowledged that CMS cannot definitively determine the extent to which reporting is incomplete.

Reported Non-DSH Supplemental Payments Were over $8 Billion Higher during 2010 Than during 2006, and New and Modified Supplemental Payments Were a Factor in the Increase

The 39 states that separately reported non-DSH supplemental payments during either 2006 or 2010 (or both) reported an increase of $8.1 billion in non-DSH supplemental payments during this period.[29] Most of this increase was from 15 states that reported during both years, and most of the reported increase was for inpatient hospital services. However, because of the potential for underreporting of supplemental payments for one or both years, the extent of the actual increase and the contributing factors cannot be quantified. Our examination of information from CMS and from public sources about changes in 11 judgmentally selected states indicates that some states were making new and modified non-DSH supplemental payments during this period, contributing to the reported increase. Changes in reporting also contributed to the increase.

[29]In constant dollars, we estimate that the $6.3 billion in non-DSH supplemental payments reported by states in 2006 would have totaled $7 billion in 2010, or an increase of about $700 million. This estimate is based on the Bureau of Economic Analysis price index for Health Care Services, downloaded June 5, 2012.

States Reported $8.1 Billion More in Non-DSH Supplemental Payments during 2010 Than during 2006

The 39 states that separately reported non-DSH supplemental payments during either 2006 or 2010, or during both years, together reported $8.1 billion more in non-DSH supplemental payments during 2010 than 2006.[30] Nineteen states separately reported some non-DSH supplemental payments during both years, with 15 of those states reporting more for these payments during 2010 and 4 of those states reporting less for these payments during 2010. Eleven states reported non-DSH supplemental payments separately only during 2010, and 9 states reported non-DSH supplemental payments separately only during 2006. (See fig. 4 and table 1.) Most of the $8.1 billion increase was from the 15 states that separately reported non-DSH supplemental payments during both years, with higher non-DSH supplemental payments reported during 2010. The increase in these states ranged from $1 million (Washington) to $2.3 billion (Texas). For the 4 states that separately reported lower non-DSH supplemental payments during 2010, the decrease ranged from $12 million (Oklahoma) to $608 million (North Carolina).

---

[30]There were 12 states that did not separately report non-DSH supplemental payments during either 2006 or 2010.

GAO-12-694 Supplemental Medicaid Payments

Figure 4: States' Separate Reporting of Non-DSH Supplemental Payments during Fiscal Years 2006 and 2010

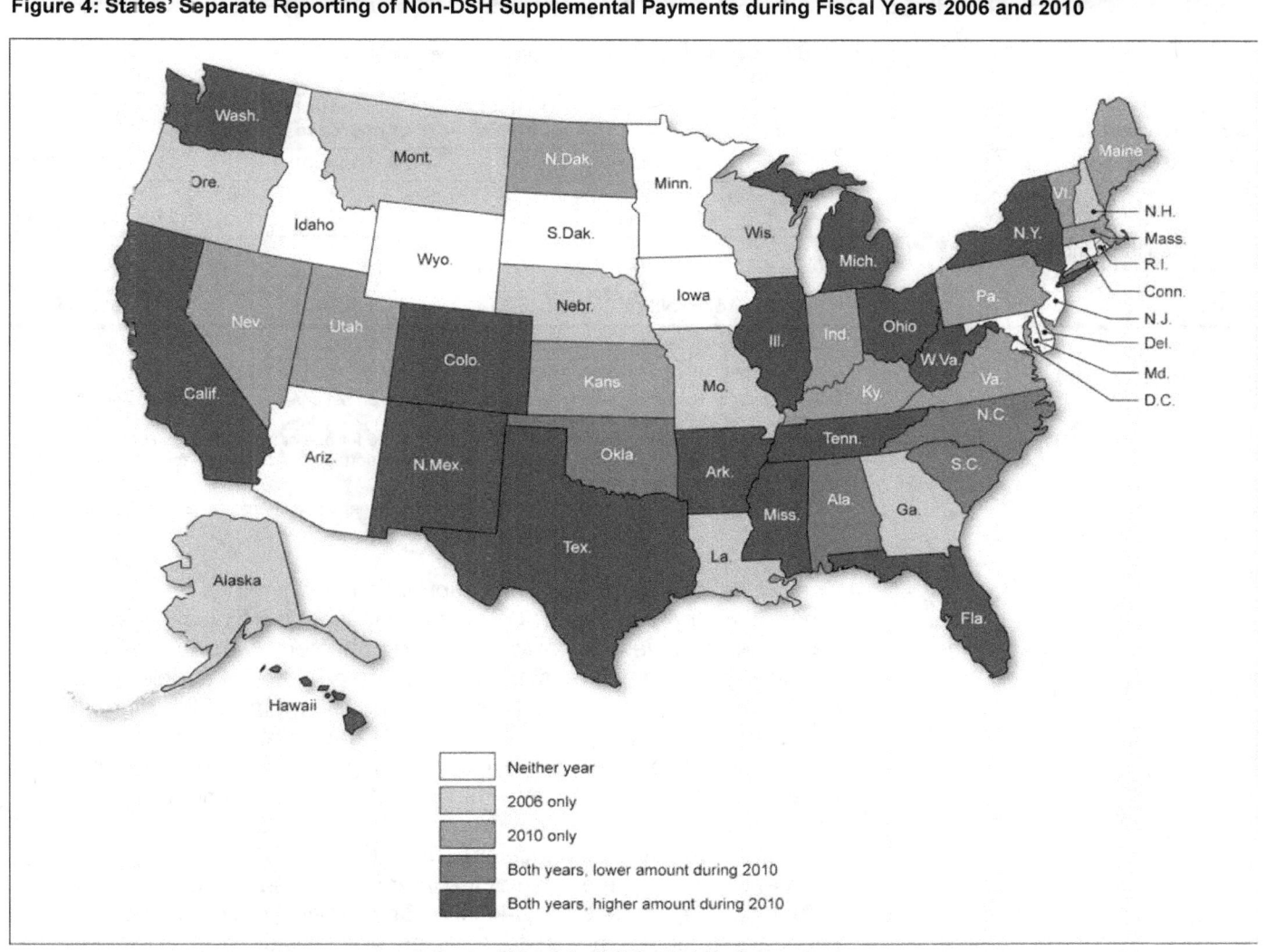

Sources: GAO analysis of CMS files (data); Map Resources (map).

Note: Puerto Rico and the U.S. territories that operate Medicaid programs are not included on this map because they did not report any supplemental Medicaid payments during 2010.

Table 1: States' Separate Reporting of Non-DSH Supplemental Payments during 2006 and 2010, by Relative Payment Amount

State reporting category	Reported higher payments during 2010		Reported lower payments during 2010		Total	
	Number of states	Amount of increase	Number of states	Amount of decrease	Number of states	Net change
Reported during 2006 and 2010[a]	15	$8.5 billion	4	($0.9 billion)	19	$7.7 billion
Reported during 2010, but not during 2006	11	$1.1 billion	NA	$0	11	$1.1 billion
Did not report during 2010, but did report during 2006	NA	$0	9	($0.7 billion)	9	($0.7 billion)
Total	26	$9.6 billion	13	($1.5 billion)	39[b]	$8.1 billion

Source: GAO analysis of CMS-64 expenditure data.

Note: Values do not sum because of rounding.

[a]Listed amounts for increases and decreases are based on net changes within states. Some states' reported non-DSH supplemental payments were higher in 2010 than in 2006 for one or more categories of service, but were lower in 2010 than in 2006 for one or more other categories of service, and some states that reported payments in both years reported $0 in payments for some categories of service in one of the years.

[b]Twelve states did not separately report non-DSH supplemental payments during either 2006 or 2010.

The largest change in non-DSH supplemental payments separately reported during 2006 and 2010 was for inpatient hospital services. The net increase in these separately reported payments was $6.3 billion, and the number of states that separately reported non-DSH supplemental payments for inpatient hospital services increased from 23 during 2006 to 27 during 2010. (App. III lists the amounts each state reported separately for non-DSH supplemental payments during 2006 and 2010 and the categories of service for which they reported these payments.)

Because of the potential underreporting of non-DSH supplemental payments during one or both of the years examined, the extent of the actual increase cannot be quantified. On the basis of some reports, Medicaid spending on hospital services is increasing, and growth in non-DSH supplemental payments has been cited as a contributing factor. A January 2012 article on the growth in U.S. health spending found that while overall Medicaid spending growth slowed in 2010, Medicaid spending growth on hospital services increased in 2010 compared to

2009.[31] The researchers attributed the growth in Medicaid spending for hospital services, in part, to a large amount of non-DSH supplemental payments reported during the last quarter of calendar year 2010. A March 2012 report by the Medicaid and CHIP Payment and Access Commission found that states reported over $23 billion in non-DSH supplemental payments for hospital services during 2011.[32]

New and Modified Supplemental Payments Contributed to Increases in Reported Payments

Information from CMS and from public sources about changes in 11 judgmentally selected states suggests that some increases from 2006 to 2010 in reported non-DSH supplemental payments were due to increases in payments states made after establishing new non-DSH supplemental payments or increasing their existing non-DSH supplemental payments. The available information suggests that changes to existing payments also resulted in some decreases from 2006 to 2010 in reported non-DSH supplemental payments, including, for example, when states terminated non-DSH supplemental payments.

In recent years, states have submitted and received approval to implement new non-DSH supplemental payments, according to CMS officials. Available information, maintained by CMS and derived from state Medicaid plans from 11 selected states, indicates that new or modified supplemental payments made by states contributed to increased non-DSH supplemental payments. For example:

- Illinois reported $1.4 billion more for non-DSH supplemental payments for inpatient hospital services during 2010 than during 2006. From 2006 through 2010, Illinois established new non-DSH supplemental payments for inpatient hospital services and also modified several existing payments for these services. Taken together, these new and modified payments were estimated to result in an increase in Illinois's

---

[31]Researchers compared health care spending growth for calendar years 2009 and 2010. They found that Medicaid spending growth slowed from 8.9 percent in 2009 to 7.2 percent in 2010, whereas Medicaid spending for hospital services grew from 10.4 percent in 2009 to 11.2 percent in 2010. Anne B. Martin, David Lassman, Benjamin Washington, Aaron Catlin, and the National Health Expenditure Accounts Team, "Growth in U.S. Health Spending Remained Slow in 2010; Health Share of Gross Domestic Product Was Unchanged from 2009," *Health Affairs*, vol. 31, no. 1 (2012).

[32]Medicaid and CHIP Payment and Access Commission, *Report to the Congress on Medicaid and CHIP* (Washington, D.C.: 2012).

supplemental payments for inpatient services by about $1.2 billion during fiscal year 2010.

- Colorado reported $411 million more for non-DSH supplemental payments for inpatient and outpatient hospital services during 2010 than during 2006. Colorado established a set of new non-DSH supplemental payments for inpatient and outpatient hospital services. These supplemental payments were to a variety of hospital types, including rural hospitals, hospitals with neonatal intensive care units, and state teaching hospitals. Effective on July 1, 2009, these new payments were estimated to result in an increase in payments of about $300 million during fiscal year 2010.

- Arkansas reported $173 million more for non-DSH supplemental payments for inpatient hospital services during 2010 than during 2006. Arkansas made new non-DSH supplemental payments for inpatient hospital services provided by private hospitals, and it also modified existing non-DSH supplemental payments for inpatient hospital services. Arkansas's new supplemental payments, effective July 1, 2009, were estimated to increase the state's supplemental payments for inpatient services by about $110 million during fiscal year 2010.

- South Carolina reported $39 million for non-DSH supplemental payments for nursing facility services during 2010, but did not report making such payments during 2006. South Carolina had suspended certain non-DSH supplemental payments for nursing facility services prior to fiscal year 2006, but it reinstated these payments, effective on October 1, 2008, with a slight change to payment qualification criteria. Reinstating these payments was estimated to increase payments by about $25 million during fiscal year 2010.

According to the available information about changes in these 11 judgmentally selected states, some states' non-DSH supplemental payments decreased from 2006 to 2010 because they terminated supplemental payments or made changes to their Medicaid programs that reduced supplemental payments. For example:

- North Carolina reported $607 million less in non-DSH supplemental payments for inpatient and outpatient hospital services in 2010 than in 2006. According to CMS, North Carolina discontinued making non-DSH supplemental payments to non-state government hospitals, effective on October 1, 2006. Discontinuation of these payments for inpatient and outpatient hospitals would have resulted in a reduction in payments.

- Georgia reported $221 million less in non-DSH supplemental payments for inpatient and outpatient hospital services in 2010 than in 2006. Georgia implemented a managed care program in 2007, and according to CMS, the state estimated that its supplemental payments (which generally can only be made for services provided on a fee-for-service basis) were reduced by more than $100 million per year as a result.

- Missouri reported paying $70 million in non-DSH supplemental payments for inpatient hospital services during 2006 and did not report making such payments during fiscal year 2010. According to CMS, the state reported that it did not make non-DSH supplemental payments for inpatient services during fiscal year 2010 because the State General Assembly did not approve funding for such payments.

Changes in State Reporting Also Contributed to Differences in Reported Supplemental Payments

Changes in state reporting of non-DSH supplemental payments also contributed to differences in amounts between 2006 and 2010. In some cases, an apparent increase in non-DSH supplemental payments was due, at least in part, to more complete reporting of non-DSH supplemental payments in 2010 than in 2006. For example:

- Pennsylvania reported $0 for non-DSH supplemental payments during 2006 and $410 million for non-DSH supplemental payments for nursing facility services during 2010, for an apparent increase of $410 million in supplemental payments. However, Pennsylvania made, but did not separately report, non-DSH supplemental payments for nursing home services during 2006.

- South Carolina reported $0 for non-DSH supplemental payments for physician and surgical services during 2006 and $46 million for non-DSH supplemental payments for these services during 2010, for an apparent increase of $46 million in supplemental payments. However, CMS told us that South Carolina paid $43 million for non-DSH supplemental payments for physician and surgical services during 2006, so the actual increase in payments for these services from 2006 to 2010 was $3 million, not $46 million.

In contrast, an apparent decrease in some states' non-DSH supplemental payments was due, at least in part, to not reporting these payments separately during 2010. For example, as noted above, Georgia made, but did not separately report, non-DSH supplemental payments during 2010. States that did not separately report payments during 2010, but did separately report them in 2006, created the appearance of decreases in non-DSH supplemental payments.

Concluding Observations

Medicaid supplemental payments can help ensure that providers make important services available to Medicaid beneficiaries. However, the transparency and accountability of these often very large payments have been lacking. Although CMS has instituted new reporting procedures for, and more complete reporting of, non-DSH supplemental payments, the exact amount of these payments is still not known because not all states have provided complete information as CMS requested during 2010. Nevertheless, as reporting of non-DSH supplemental payments becomes more complete, the significance of these payments, in terms of cost, growth, and contribution to total Medicaid payments for those providers receiving them, is becoming clearer. Identifying and monitoring Medicaid supplemental payments and ensuring that they, along with regular Medicaid payments, are consistent with federal requirements are complex tasks that will require continued vigilance by CMS. Ongoing federal efforts to improve the completeness of reporting of Medicaid supplemental payments are important for effective oversight and to better understand these payments' role in financing Medicaid services.

Agency Comments

We provided a draft of this report to HHS for review. HHS stated that HHS and CMS will continue their ongoing efforts to improve states' reporting of Medicaid supplemental payments. HHS's letter is reprinted in appendix IV.

As agreed with your offices, unless you publicly announce the contents of this report earlier, we plan no further distribution until 30 days from the report date. At that time, we will send copies to the Secretary of Health and Human Services, the Administrator of the Centers for Medicare & Medicaid Services, and other interested parties. In addition, the report will be available at no charge on the GAO website at http://www.gao.gov.

If you or your staff members have any questions, please contact me at (202) 512-7114 or iritanik@gao.gov. Contact points for our Offices of Congressional Relations and Public Affairs may be found on the last page of this report. Major contributors to this report are listed in appendix V.

Katherine M. Iritani
Director, Health Care

Appendix I: Scope and Methodology

This appendix provides information about our analyses of reported supplemental Medicaid expenditures and our analyses of information from selected states. Supplemental Medicaid payments include Disproportionate Share Hospital (DSH) payments to hospitals and other supplemental payments to hospitals or other providers, which we refer to as non-DSH supplemental payments. To determine what supplemental Medicaid payments states reported during fiscal year 2010 and how non-DSH supplemental payments reported during 2010 compared with those reported during 2006, we obtained and analyzed data about the Medicaid expenditures states reported during these 2 years.[1] To examine reasons for differences between 2006 and 2010 in reported non-DSH supplemental payments, and to obtain additional information about states' reports of these payments, we obtained information from the Centers for Medicare & Medicaid Services (CMS) and public sources about non-DSH supplemental payments in a nongeneralizable, judgmental sample of 11 states. In addition, we reviewed relevant federal laws, regulations, and guidance; our prior work on supplemental Medicaid payments; and other relevant documentation. We also interviewed officials from CMS.

Reported Expenditures

To determine what Medicaid payments states reported, we examined data from the standardized expenditure reports states submit to CMS on a quarterly basis using form CMS-64. States have 30 days after the end of a quarter to submit this form and must certify that the data are correct to the best of their knowledge. CMS reviews these reports and works with states to resolve any questions before certifying them as final. CMS transfers the certified, finalized data into a Financial Management Report (FMR) and makes annual data available on its website. CMS allows states to make adjustments to their prior CMS-64 submissions for up to 2 years. The annual FMR incorporates adjustments reported by the states by applying reported adjustments to the fiscal year during which they are reported, even if an adjustment corrects expenditures reported during an earlier fiscal year.

Expenditures reported during fiscal year 2010. We obtained fiscal year 2010 FMR data from CMS on December 22, 2011. These data reflected adjustments to expenditures reported by states on the quarterly reports filed during fiscal year 2010 and included states' reported total Medicaid

---

[1]Throughout this report, the term fiscal year refers to the federal fiscal year.

expenditures, DSH expenditures, and any non-DSH expenditures the states reported separately from their other expenditures. Fiscal year 2010 was the most recent year for which certified data were available from all 50 states and the District of Columbia.[2] To assess the reliability of the fiscal year 2010 data, we reviewed the steps CMS took to ensure the accuracy of expenditure data and we examined the data for outliers or other unusual values, which we discussed with CMS officials. We determined that the data were sufficiently reliable to describe the expenditures reported by the states during fiscal year 2010, although as discussed in this report, we found that states' separate reporting of non-DSH supplemental payments was incomplete.

Expenditures reported during fiscal year 2006. We obtained data about expenditures reported during fiscal year 2006 as part of work we reported in 2008.[3] For that work, we obtained reported DSH payments from CMS's FMR for fiscal year 2006, which included adjustments reported by states for prior years. To obtain data about non-DSH supplemental payments, we extracted expenditure data that had been reported on a section of the CMS expenditure report—the form CMS-64.9I—that states were to use for informational purposes during 2006 to identify non-DSH supplemental payments made under Medicaid's Upper Payment Limit regulations.[4] We adjusted these data to reflect adjustments states reported through their CMS-64.9I entries during fiscal year 2006 and through October 5, 2007. As described in our 2008 report, our assessment of the reliability of the fiscal year 2006 data included review of the steps CMS took to ensure the accuracy of expenditure data submitted to the Medicaid Budget and Expenditure System, comparison to data we obtained from a nongeneralizable sample of 5 states, and

---

[2]Data from Puerto Rico and the U.S. territories that operate Medicaid programs (American Samoa, Guam, the Northern Mariana Islands, and the U.S. Virgin Islands), which did not report supplemental Medicaid payments during fiscal year 2010, were not necessarily complete.

[3]See GAO-08-614.

[4]For expenditures incurred during fiscal year 2006, states received federal matching funds for non-DSH payments based on the information they provided on sections of the CMS-64 other than the CMS-64.9I. Specifically, reimbursement for non-DSH supplemental payments was normally based on the CMS-64.9 base form, on which states reported regular payments and non-DSH supplemental payments together. Reimbursement for supplemental payments made under Medicaid demonstrations was based on CMS-64.9 waiver forms. Specific reporting requirements for supplemental payments made under demonstration waivers varied.

comparison to similar data published by the Urban Institute.[5] We determined that the data were sufficiently reliable to describe the expenditures identified by the states during fiscal year 2006, although as we discussed in our earlier report, we concluded that states' separate reporting of non-DSH supplemental payments was incomplete.

Our analyses of reported DSH and non-DSH payments included identification of state-by-state and nationwide expenditures for DSH and non-DSH supplemental payments in both absolute (dollar amount) and relative (percentage) terms. DSH payments can be made to hospitals for traditional inpatient and outpatient services and to mental health facilities for inpatient and outpatient mental health services; we examined reported payments to both types of hospitals. Non-DSH supplemental payments can be made for various categories of service (such as inpatient hospital services or physician and surgical services) provided by hospitals or other types of providers (such as nursing homes or intermediate care facilities); we examined payments for specific categories of services.

Some states may not have separately reported all of their non-DSH supplemental payments during 2006 or 2010. We did not quantify the extent to which states did not separately report their supplemental payments. Therefore, we may not be capturing the full amount of states' non-DSH supplemental payments or the degree to which these payments have changed over time. We did not examine whether changes in non-DSH supplemental payments were associated with changes in states' regular Medicaid payments.

Information from Selected States

To examine reasons for differences between 2006 and 2010 in reported non-DSH supplemental payments, and to obtain additional information about states' reports of these payments, we obtained information from CMS and public sources about non-DSH supplemental payments in a judgmental sample of 11 states selected to include a mix of relevant characteristics. We selected a nongeneralizable sample of states, including some that separately reported non-DSH supplemental payments (1) in fiscal year 2006, but not 2010 (Georgia and Missouri); (2) in fiscal year 2010, but not 2006 (Maine, Massachusetts, and

---

[5]See T. A. Coughlin, S. Zuckerman, and J. McFeeters, "Restoring Fiscal Integrity to Medicaid Financing? Some Progress Has Been Made in Reforming Medicaid Financing, Yet Problems Persist," *Health Affairs*, vol. 26, no. 5 (2007).

Pennsylvania); and (3) both (Arkansas, Colorado, Illinois, North Carolina, South Carolina, and Texas). These states differed in absolute and relative changes in reported non-DSH supplemental payments and changes in categories of service for which payments were reported. The information we used to select states included published information as well as preliminary information from CMS.[6] (For more information about non-DSH supplemental payments made by these states in 2006 and 2010, see app. III.)

For each of our selected states, we asked CMS to provide us with documentation, such as state plan amendments, that could shed light on observed differences from 2006 to 2010 in reported non-DSH supplemental payments. We reviewed this information, along with information from other public sources (such as states' websites) to identify possible reasons for changes in reported payments and to develop rough estimates of the financial impact of planned changes. The state plan amendments states submit when proposing new supplemental payments, or modifications to existing payments, include an estimate of the financial impact of the state plan amendment. This estimate is intended to reflect the impact of the state plan amendment as a whole, even if the amendment covers several changes. CMS officials told us that these estimates are the best available estimates of the financial impact of changes states make to their state plans.

We did not attempt to develop a full, dollar-by-dollar explanation of any state's changes from 2006 to 2010 in reported amounts of non-DSH supplemental payments. We did not determine the accuracy of states' estimates of the financial impact of their state plan amendments. Information from our judgmental sample of 11 states cannot be generalized to other states.

---

[6]Expenditure data from fiscal year 2010 had not been finalized at the time we made our selections.

Appendix II: Supplemental Medicaid Payments Reported during 2010

This appendix provides state-by-state and nationwide information about the DSH and non-DSH supplemental Medicaid payments reported during fiscal year 2010 by the states and the District of Columbia.[1]

- Table 2 shows states' reported Medicaid payments, their DSH and non-DSH supplemental payments, the federal share of DSH and non-DSH supplemental payments, and the percentage of the state Medicaid payments that was for DSH and non-DSH supplemental payments.

- Table 3 shows states' reported DSH payments, including payments for traditional and mental health hospitals (as dollar amounts and as a percentage of the state DSH payments), total DSH payments, and total DSH payments as a percentage of the national total for DSH payments.

- Table 4 shows states' reported non-DSH supplemental payments, including the amounts states reported for certain categories of service (as dollar amounts and as a percentage of the state non-DSH supplemental payments), total non-DSH supplemental payments, and total non-DSH supplemental payments as a percentage of the national total for non-DSH supplemental payments. The six categories of service listed are those for which CMS requested information— inpatient hospital services, outpatient hospital services, nursing facility services, physician and surgical services, other practitioners' services, and intermediate care facility services.

- Tables 5 through 10 provide additional information about states' reported Medicaid payments for the six categories of service for which CMS obtained information about non-DSH supplemental payments— inpatient hospital services, outpatient hospital services, nursing facility services, physician and surgical services, other practitioners' services, and intermediate care facility services. For each of these six categories, the tables provide the states' reported Medicaid payments, non-DSH supplemental payments, the federal share of the non-DSH payments, and the percentage of the state Medicaid payments for this category that was for non-DSH supplemental payments.

---

[1]Puerto Rico and the U.S. territories that operate Medicaid programs—American Samoa, Guam, the Northern Mariana Islands, and the U.S. Virgin Islands—did not report supplemental Medicaid payments during fiscal year 2010.

Table 2: State Supplemental Medicaid Payments Reported during Fiscal Year 2010 as a Percentage of Total Reported State Medicaid Payments

Dollars in millions

State	Total state Medicaid payments[a]	DSH supplemental payments			Non-DSH supplemental payments		
		Total	Federal share	Total as percentage of state's Medicaid payments	Total	Federal share	Total as percentage of state's Medicaid payments
Alabama	$4,709	$467	$318	10	$227	$176	5
Alaska	1,208	25	13	2	0	0	0
Arizona	9,380	28	19	<1	0	0	0
Arkansas	3,881	61	44	2	292	237	8
California	41,643	2,157	1,079	5	1,786	1,160	4
Colorado	4,028	200	100	5	682	418	17
Connecticut	5,528	269	134	5	0	0	0
Delaware	1,287	6	3	<1	0	0	0
District of Columb a	1,772	67	47	4	0	0	0
Florida	17,262	376	207	2	1,485	1,004	9
Georgia	7,711	435	283	6	0	0	0
Hawaii	1,361	8	4	1	22	15	2
Idaho	1,345	24	17	2	0	0	0
Illinois	15,196	565	283	4	2,659	1,646	18
Indiana	5,879	156	100	3	178	134	3
Iowa	3,047	49	31	2	0	0	0
Kansas	2,408	68	41	3	54	38	2
Kentucky	5,522	211	150	4	77	62	1
Louisiana	6,720	791	521	12	0	0	0
Maine	2,266	50	32	2	57	43	3
Maryland	7,012	113	56	2	0	0	0
Massachusetts	11,595	0	0	0	213	131	2
Michigan	11,556	377	238	3	914	669	8
Minnesota	7,496	109	55	1	0	0	0
Mississippi	4,106	208	158	5	434	368	11
Missouri	7,994	739	476	9	0	0	0
Montana	928	17	12	2	0	0	0
Nebraska	1,595	48	29	3	0	0	0
Nevada	1,505	95	48	6	39	25	3
New Hampshire	1,319	230	115	17	0	0	0

Dollars in millions

State	Total state Medicaid payments[a]	DSH supplemental payments				Non-DSH supplemental payments		
		Total	Federal share	Total as percentage of state's Medicaid payments		Total	Federal share	Total as percentage of state's Medicaid payments
New Jersey	10,163	1,340	670	13		0	0	0
New Mexico	3,457	29	21	1		100	80	3
New York	50,453	3,117	1,559	6		513	316	1
North Carolina	10,319	468	305	5		218	163	2
North Dakota	682	2	1	<1		8	6	1
Ohio	15,122	656	409	4		155	114	1
Oklahoma	3,862	40	26	1		16	12	<1
Oregon	3,973	54	34	1		0	0	0
Pennsylvania	18,634	844	462	5		410	270	2
Rhode Island	1,912	125	66	7		0	0	0
South Carolina	4,992	418	294	8		145	116	3
South Dakota	775	1	<1	<1		0	0	0
Tennessee	8,441	140	92	2		444	392	5
Texas	26,331	1,688	992	6		3,099	2,184	12
Utah	1,687	27	19	2		17	14	1
Vermont	1,247	37	21	3		<1	<1	<1
Virginia	6,408	199	99	3		29	17	<1
Washington	6,989	368	184	5		11	7	<1
West Virginia	2,539	74	55	3		137	112	5
Wisconsin	6,432	4	2	<1		0	0	0
Wyoming	530	1	<1	<1		0	0	0
Total	$383,368[b]	$17,581	$9,925	4.59		$14,420	$9,928	3.76

Source: GAO analysis of CMS-64 expenditure data.

Notes: Amounts represent payments reported during federal fiscal year 2010 and may include adjustments (positive or negative) to payments made during prior fiscal years. CMS provided these data to GAO on December 22, 2011. When a value was greater than 0, but did not round to $1 million or 1 percent, the cell includes the entry "<1."

[a]Total state Medicaid payments include both the state and federal share of payments and include all payments made by states to providers, including DSH and non-DSH payments as well as regular payments. They do not include expenditures for program administration.

[b]The nationwide total for state Medicaid payments includes about $1,160 million in payments reported by Puerto Rico and the U.S. territories.

Table 3: DSH Supplemental Payments for Traditional Hospital and Mental Health Facility Services Reported during Fiscal Year 2010

Dollars in millions

State	DSH payments (percentage of state DSH total)		Total state DSH payments	State total as percentage of national DSH total
	Traditional hospital services[a]	Mental health facility services		
Alabama	$464 (99)	$3 (1)	**$467**	3
Alaska	11 (45)	14 (55)	**$25**	<1
Arizona	0 (0)	28 (100)	**$28**	<1
Arkansas	60 (99)	1 (1)	**$61**	<1
California	2,157 (100)	0 (0)	**$2,157**	12
Colorado	200 (100)	0 (0)	**$200**	1
Connecticut	160 (60)	109 (40)	**$269**	2
Delaware	0 (0)	6 (100)	**$6**	<1
District of Columbia	65 (97)	2 (3)	**$67**	<1
Florida	254 (68)	122 (32)	**$376**	2
Georgia	435 (100)	0 (0)	**$435**	2
Hawaii	8 (100)	0 (0)	**$8**	<1
Idaho	24 (100)	0 (0)	**$24**	<1
Illinois	475 (84)	89 (16)	**$565**	3
Indiana	58 (37)	98 (63)	**$156**	1
Iowa	49 (100)	0 (0)	**$49**	<1
Kansas	45 (66)	23 (34)	**$68**	<1
Kentucky	174 (82)	37 (18)	**$211**	1
Louisiana	682 (86)	108 (14)	**$791**	4
Maine	0 (0)	50 (100)	**$50**	<1
Maryland	61 (54)	52 (46)	**$113**	1
Massachusetts	0 (0)	0 (0)	**$0**	0
Michigan	283 (75)	94 (25)	**$377**	2
Minnesota	109 (100)	<1 (<1)	**$109**	1
Mississippi	208 (100)	0 (0)	**$208**	1
Missouri	546 (74)	193 (26)	**$739**	4
Montana	17 (100)	0 (0)	**$17**	<1
Nebraska	55 (114)	-7 (-14)	**$48**	<1
Nevada	95 (100)	0 (0)	**$95**	1
New Hampshire	195 (85)	35 (15)	**$230**	1

Dollars in millions

State	DSH payments (percentage of state DSH total)		Total state DSH payments	State total as percentage of national DSH total
	Traditional hospital services[a]	Mental health facility services		
New Jersey	983 (73)	357 (27)	**$1,340**	8
New Mexico	29 (99)	<1 (1)	**$29**	<1
New York	2,714 (87)	403 (13)	**$3,117**	18
North Carolina	313 (67)	154 (33)	**$468**	3
North Dakota	1 (43)	1 (57)	**$2**	<1
Ohio	563 (86)	93 (14)	**$656**	4
Oklahoma	37 (92)	3 (8)	**$40**	<1
Oregon	34 (63)	20 (37)	**$54**	<1
Pennsylvania	518 (61)	326 (39)	**$844**	5
Rhode Island	125 (100)	0 (0)	**$125**	1
South Carolina	370 (88)	49 (12)	**$418**	2
South Dakota	0 (0)	1 (100)	**$1**	<1
Tennessee	140 (100)	0 (0)	**$140**	1
Texas	1,396 (83)	293 (17)	**$1,688**	10
Utah	26 (97)	1 (3)	**$27**	<1
Vermont	37 (100)	0 (0)	**$37**	<1
Virginia	192 (97)	6 (3)	**$199**	1
Washington	242 (66)	126 (34)	**$368**	2
West Virginia	55 (74)	19 (26)	**$74**	<1
Wisconsin	4 (100)	0 (0)	**$4**	<1
Wyoming	1 (100)	0 (0)	**$1**	<1
Total	**$14,669 (83.44)**	**$2,912 (16.56)**	**$17,581**	**100**

Source: GAO analysis of CMS-64 expenditure data.

Notes: Amounts represent payments reported during federal fiscal year 2010 and may include adjustments (positive or negative) to payments made during prior fiscal years. CMS provided these data to GAO on December 22, 2011. When a value was greater than 0, but did not round to $1 million or 1 percent, the cell includes the entry "<1."

[a]Traditional inpatient and outpatient services include services that are furnished in a hospital for the care and treatment of inpatients and outpatients, other than services provided in mental health facilities. See 42 C.F.R. §§ 440.10, 440.20 (2011).

Table 4: Non-DSH Supplemental Payments Reported during Fiscal Year 2010 by Category of Service

Dollars in millions

State	Non-DSH supplemental payments (percentage of total state non-DSH payments)[a]						Total state non-DSH supplemental payments	State total as percentage of national non-DSH total
	Inpatient hospital services	Outpatient hospital services	Nursing facility services	Physician and surgical services	Other practitioners' services[b]	Intermediate care facility services[c]		
Alabama	$210 (92)	$17 (8)	$0 (0)	$0 (0)	$0 (0)	$0 (0)	$227	2
Alaska	0 (0)	0 (0)	0 (0)	0 (0)	0 (0)	0 (0)	$0	0
Arizona	0 (0)	0 (0)	0 (0)	0 (0)	0 (0)	0 (0)	$0	0
Arkansas	236 (81)	46 (16)	0 (0)	10 (3)	0 (0)	0 (0)	$292	2
California	1,668 (93)	96 (5)	21 (1)	0 (0)	0 (0)	0 (0)	$1,786	12
Colorado	417 (61)	132 (19)	119 (17)	15 (2)	0 (0)	0 (0)	$682	5
Connecticut	0 (0)	0 (0)	0 (0)	0 (0)	0 (0)	0 (0)	$0	0
Delaware	0 (0)	0 (0)	0 (0)	0 (0)	0 (0)	0 (0)	$0	0
District of Columbia	0 (0)	0 (0)	0 (0)	0 (0)	0 (0)	0 (0)	$0	0
Florida	1,334 (90)	0 (0)	14 (1)	137 (9)	0 (0)	0 (0)	$1,485	10
Georgia	0 (0)	0 (0)	0 (0)	0 (0)	0 (0)	0 (0)	$0	0
Hawaii	18 (83)	4 (17)	0 (0)	0 (0)	0 (0)	0 (0)	$22	<1
Idaho	0 (0)	0 (0)	0 (0)	0 (0)	0 (0)	0 (0)	$0	0
Illinois	1,923 (72)	736 (28)	0 (0)	0 (0)	0 (0)	0 (0)	$2,659	18
Indiana	43 (24)	0 (0)	88 (50)	47 (27)	0 (0)	0 (0)	$178	1
Iowa	0 (0)	0 (0)	0 (0)	0 (0)	0 (0)	0 (0)	$0	0
Kansas	20 (37)	18 (33)	0 (0)	16 (29)	<1 (1)	0 (0)	$54	<1
Kentucky	54 (69)	0 (0)	<1 (1)	23 (30)	0 (0)	0 (0)	$77	1
Louisiana	0 (0)	0 (0)	0 (0)	0 (0)	0 (0)	0 (0)	$0	0
Maine	28 (48)	26 (46)	0 (0)	3 (5)	1 (1)	0 (0)	$57	<1
Maryland	0 (0)	0 (0)	0 (0)	0 (0)	0 (0)	0 (0)	$0	0
Massachusetts	46 (21)	167 (79)	0 (0)	0 (0)	0 (0)	0 (0)	$213	1
Michigan	428 (47)	116 (13)	306 (33)	64 (7)	0 (0)	0 (0)	$914	6
Minnesota	0 (0)	0 (0)	0 (0)	0 (0)	0 (0)	0 (0)	$0	0
Mississippi	434 (100)	0 (0)	0 (0)	0 (0)	0 (0)	0 (0)	$434	3
Missouri	0 (0)	0 (0)	0 (0)	0 (0)	0 (0)	0 (0)	$0	0
Montana	0 (0)	0 (0)	0 (0)	0 (0)	0 (0)	0 (0)	$0	0
Nebraska	0 (0)	0 (0)	0 (0)	0 (0)	0 (0)	0 (0)	$0	0
Nevada	35 (90)	0 (0)	0 (0)	4 (10)	0 (0)	0 (0)	$39	<1

Dollars in millions

State	Inpatient hospital services	Outpatient hospital services	Nursing facility services	Physician and surgical services	Other practitioners' services[b]	Intermediate care facility services[c]	Total state non-DSH supplemental payments	State total as percentage of national non-DSH total
New Hampshire	0 (0)	0 (0)	0 (0)	0 (0)	0 (0)	0 (0)	$0	0
New Jersey	0 (0)	0 (0)	0 (0)	0 (0)	0 (0)	0 (0)	$0	0
New Mexico	96 (96)	0 (0)	0 (0)	4 (4)	0 (0)	0 (0)	$100	1
New York	45 (9)	425 (83)	44 (9)	0 (0)	0 (0)	0 (0)	$513	4
North Carolina	218 (100)	0 (0)	0 (0)	0 (0)	0 (0)	0 (0)	$218	2
North Dakota	4 (47)	0 (0)	0 (0)	0 (0)	0 (0)	4 (53)	$8	<1
Ohio	155 (100)	0 (0)	0 (0)	0 (0)	0 (0)	0 (0)	$155	1
Oklahoma	16 (100)	0 (0)	0 (0)	<1 (<1)	0 (0)	0 (0)	$16	<1
Oregon	0 (0)	0 (0)	0 (0)	0 (0)	0 (0)	0 (0)	$0	0
Pennsylvania	0 (0)	0 (0)	410 (100)	0 (0)	0 (0)	0 (0)	$410	3
Rhode Island	0 (0)	0 (0)	0 (0)	0 (0)	0 (0)	0 (0)	$0	0
South Carolina	36 (25)	24 (16)	39 (27)	46 (32)	0 (0)	0 (0)	$145	1
South Dakota	0 (0)	0 (0)	0 (0)	0 (0)	0 (0)	0 (0)	$0	0
Tennessee	444 (100)	0 (0)	0 (0)	0 (0)	0 (0)	0 (0)	$444	3
Texas	3,050 (98)	4 (<1)	0 (0)	45 (1)	0 (0)	0 (0)	$3,099	21
Utah	0 (0)	0 (0)	0 (0)	17 (100)	0 (0)	0 (0)	$17	<1
Vermont	0 (0)	0 (0)	<1 (100)	0 (0)	0 (0)	0 (0)	<$1	<1
Virginia	1 (4)	0 (0)	4 (14)	29 (100)	0 (0)	-5 (-17)	$29	<1
Washington	<1 (1)	0 (0)	11 (103)	0 (0)	0 (0)	<0 (-4)	$11	<1
West Virginia	74 (55)	0 (0)	0 (0)	62 (45)	0 (0)	0 (0)	$137	1
Wisconsin	0 (0)	0 (0)	0 (0)	0 (0)	0 (0)	0 (0)	$0	0
Wyoming	0 (0)	0 (0)	0 (0)	0 (0)	0 (0)	0 (0)	$0	0
Total	$11,031 (76.50)	$1,811 (12.56)	$1,056 (7.32)	$522 (3.62)	$1 (0.01)	$-1 (-0.01)	$14,420	100

Source: GAO analysis of CMS-64 expenditure data.

Notes: Amounts represent payments reported during federal fiscal year 2010 and may include adjustments (positive or negative) to payments made during prior fiscal years. CMS provided these data to GAO on December 22, 2011. When a value was greater than 0, but did not round to $1 million or 1 percent, the cell includes the entry "<1." When a value was less than 0, but did not round to ($1) million or (1 percent), the cell includes the entry "<0."

[a]CMS did not ask states to report non-DSH supplemental payments for other categories of service, such as mental health facility services or clinic services.

[b]Other practitioners' services that may be covered by Medicaid vary from state to state and include health-related or remedial care or services, other than physicians' services, provided by licensed practitioners acting within the scope of practice defined under state law. For example, depending on the state, such services could be provided by chiropractors, nurse midwives, nurse practitioners, and others.

[c]Intermediate care facility services include those provided by facilities serving individuals with intellectual disabilities.

Table 5: Non-DSH Supplemental Payments for Inpatient Hospital Services Reported during Fiscal Year 2010

Dollars in millions

State	Total state Medicaid payments for inpatient hospital services[a]	Non-DSH supplemental payments for inpatient hospital services		Non-DSH supplemental payments as a percentage of state's total for inpatient hospital services
		Total	Federal share	
Alabama	$790	$210	$163	27
Alaska	185	0	0	0
Arizona	136	0	0	0
Arkansas	740	236	191	32
California	8,667	1,668	1,092	19
Colorado	975	417	257	43
Connecticut	597	0	0	0
Delaware	52	0	0	0
District of Columbia	369	0	0	0
Florida	3,956	1,334	902	34
Georgia	1,728	0	0	0
Hawaii	81	18	12	23
Idaho	228	0	0	0
Illinois	5,567	1,923	1,190	35
Indiana	366	43	32	12
Iowa	206	0	0	0
Kansas	302	20	14	7
Kentucky	1,027	54	43	5
Louisiana	2,159	0	0	0
Maine	209	28	21	13
Maryland	809	0	0	0
Massachusetts	1,129	46	28	4
Michigan	1,346	428	313	32
Minnesota	528	0	0	0
Mississippi	1,252	434	368	35
Missouri	2,220	0	0	0
Montana	164	0	0	0
Nebraska	259	0	0	0

Dollars in millions

State	Total state Medicaid payments for inpatient hospital services[a]	Non-DSH supplemental payments for inpatient hospital services		Non-DSH supplemental payments as a percentage of state's total for inpatient hospital services
		Total	Federal share	
Nevada	285	35	22	12
New Hampshire	258	0	0	0
New Jersey	1,717	0	0	0
New Mexico	460[b]	96	77	21
New York	8,781	45	28	1
North Carolina	1,983	218	163	11
North Dakota	50	4	3	8
Ohio	1,714	155	114	9
Oklahoma	934	16	12	2
Oregon	241	0	0	0
Pennsylvania	1,146	0	0	0
Rhode Island	322	0	0	0
South Carolina	1,070	36	29	3
South Dakota	155	0	0	0
Tennessee	932	444	392	48
Texas	6,629	3,050	2,150	46
Utah	360	0	0	0
Vermont	40	0	0	0
Virginia	852	1	1	<1
Washington	914	<1	<1	<1
West Virginia	293	74	62	25
Wisconsin	434	0	0	0
Wyoming	96	0	0	0
Total	$65,762[b]	$11,031	$7,678	16.77

Source: GAO analysis of CMS-64 expenditure data.

Notes: Amounts represent payments reported during federal fiscal year 2010 and may include adjustments (positive or negative) to payments made during prior fiscal years. CMS provided these data to GAO on December 22, 2011. When a value was greater than 0, but did not round to $1 million or 1 percent, the cell includes the entry "<1."

[a]Total state Medicaid payments for inpatient hospital services include both the state and federal share of payments and include all payments made by states to providers, including DSH and non-DSH payments as well as regular payments. They do not include expenditures for program administration.

[b]The nationwide total for state Medicaid payments for inpatient hospital services includes about $48 million in payments reported by Puerto Rico and the U.S. territories.

Table 6: Non-DSH Supplemental Payments for Outpatient Hospital Services Reported during Fiscal Year 2010

Dollars in millions

State	Total state Medicaid payments for outpatient hospital services[a]	Non-DSH supplemental payments for outpatient hospital services		Non-DSH supplemental payments as a percentage of state's total for outpatient hospital services
		Total	Federal share	
Alabama	$267	$17	$13	6
Alaska	108	0	0	0
Arizona	311	0	0	0
Arkansas	171	46	38	27
California	1,346	96	57	7
Colorado	305	132	81	43
Connecticut	165	0	0	0
Delaware	18	0	0	0
District of Columbia	40	0	0	0
Florida	840	0	0	0
Georgia	316	0	0	0
Hawaii	17	4	3	23
Idaho	54	0	0	0
Illinois	1,289	736	455	57
Indiana	99	0	0	0
Iowa	190	0	0	0
Kansas	56	18	12	32
Kentucky	289	0	0	0
Louisiana	424	0	0	0
Maine	215	26	20	12
Maryland	198	0	0	0
Massachusetts	837	167	103	20
Michigan	315	116	85	37
Minnesota	101	0	0	0
Mississippi	324	0	0	0
Missouri	535	0	0	0
Montana	59	0	0	0
Nebraska	92	0	0	0

Dollars in millions

State	Total state Medicaid payments for outpatient hospital services[a]	Non-DSH supplemental payments for outpatient hospital services		Non-DSH supplemental payments as a percentage of state's total for outpatient hospital services
		Total	Federal share	
Nevada	97	0	0	0
New Hampshire	75	0	0	0
New Jersey	282	0	0	0
New Mexico	104	0	0	0
New York	2,079	425	262	20
North Carolina	697	0	0	0
North Dakota	25	0	0	0
Ohio	383	0	0	0
Oklahoma	230	0	0	0
Oregon	15	0	0	0
Pennsylvania	359	0	0	0
Rhode Island	37	0	0	0
South Carolina	225	24	19	11
South Dakota	50	0	0	0
Tennessee	17	0	0	0
Texas	1,112	4	3	<1
Utah	58	0	0	0
Vermont	2	0	0	0
Virginia	135	0	0	0
Washington	244	0	0	0
West Virginia	93	0	0	0
Wisconsin	165	0	0	0
Wyoming	38	0	0	0
Total	$15,506[b]	1,811	$1,150	11.68

Source: GAO analysis of CMS-64 expenditure data.

Notes: Amounts represent payments reported during federal fiscal year 2010 and may include adjustments (positive or negative) to payments made during prior fiscal years. CMS provided these data to GAO on December 22, 2011. When a value was greater than 0, but did not round to $1 million or 1 percent, the cell includes the entry "<1."

[a]Total state Medicaid payments for outpatient hospital services include both the state and federal share of payments and include all payments made by states to providers, including non-DSH payments as well as regular payments. They do not include expenditures for program administration.

[b]The nationwide total for state Medicaid payments for outpatient hospital services includes about $5 million in payments reported by Puerto Rico and the U.S. territories.

Table 7: Non-DSH Supplemental Payments for Nursing Facility Services Reported during Fiscal Year 2010

Dollars in millions

State	Total state Medicaid payments for nursing facility services[a]	Non-DSH supplemental payments for nursing facility services		Non-DSH supplemental payments as a percentage of state's total for nursing facility services
		Total	Federal share	
Alabama	$875	$0	$0	0
Alaska	118	0	0	0
Arizona	34	0	0	0
Arkansas	615	0	0	0
California	4,268	21	11	<1
Colorado	573	119	73	21
Connecticut	1,254	0	0	0
Delaware	186	0	0	0
District of Columbia	205	0	0	0
Florida	2,786	14	9	<1
Georgia	1,133	0	0	0
Hawaii	2	0	0	0
Idaho	125	0	0	0
Illinois	1,520	0	0	0
Indiana	1,166	88	67	8
Iowa	501	0	0	0
Kansas	355	0	0	0
Kentucky	837	<1	<1	<1
Louisiana	776	0	0	0
Maine	237	0	0	0
Maryland	1,060	0	0	0
Massachusetts	1,583	0	0	0
Michigan	1,686	306	224	18
Minnesota	812	0	0	0
Mississippi	748	0	0	0
Missouri	905	0	0	0
Montana	156	0	0	0
Nebraska	314	0	0	0

Dollars in millions

| State | Total state Medicaid payments for nursing facility services[a] | Non-DSH supplemental payments for nursing facility services | | Non-DSH supplemental payments as a percentage of state's total for nursing facility services |
		Total	Federal share	
Nevada	171	0	0	0
New Hampshire	309	0	0	0
New Jersey	1,968	0	0	0
New Mexico	5	0	0	0
New York	6,852	44	27	1
North Carolina	1,228	0	0	0
North Dakota	187	0	0	0
Ohio	2,743	0	0	0
Oklahoma	508	0	0	0
Oregon	323	0	0	0
Pennsylvania	3,504	410	270	12
Rhode Island	304	0	0	0
South Carolina	571	39	31	7
South Dakota	144	0	0	0
Tennessee	624	0	0	0
Texas	2,307	0	0	0
Utah	158	0	0	0
Vermont	115	<1	<1	<1
Virginia	806	4	2	<1
Washington	576	11	7	2
West Virginia	480	0	0	0
Wisconsin	923	0	0	0
Wyoming	74	0	0	0
Total	**$49,713[b]**	**$1,056**	**$722**	**2.12**

Source: GAO analysis of CMS-64 expenditure data.

Notes: Amounts represent payments reported during federal fiscal year 2010 and may include adjustments (positive or negative) to payments made during prior fiscal years. CMS provided these data to GAO on December 22, 2011. When a value was greater than 0, but did not round to $1 million or 1 percent, the cell includes the entry "<1."

[a]Total state Medicaid payments for nursing facility services include both the state and federal share of payments and include all payments made by states to providers, including non-DSH payments as well as regular payments. They do not include expenditures for program administration.

[b]The nationwide total for state Medicaid payments for nursing facility services includes about $2 million in payments reported by Puerto Rico and the U.S. territories.

Table 8: Non-DSH Supplemental Payments for Physician and Surgical Services Reported during Fiscal Year 2010

Dollars in millions

State	Total state Medicaid payments for physician and surgical services[a]	Non-DSH supplemental payments for physician and surgical services		Non-DSH supplemental payments as a percentage of state's total for physician and surgical services
		Total	Federal share	
Alabama	$301	$0	$0	0
Alaska	94	0	0	0
Arizona	38	0	0	0
Arkansas	276	10	8	4
California	1,388	0	0	0
Colorado	272	15	8	5
Connecticut	70	0	0	0
Delaware	22	0	0	0
District of Columbia	55	0	0	0
Florida	1,089	137	93	13
Georgia	355	0	0	0
Hawaii	7	0	0	0
Idaho	100	0	0	0
Illinois	880	0	0	0
Indiana	189	47	36	25
Iowa	174	0	0	0
Kansas	97	16	11	16
Kentucky	374	23	19	6
Louisiana	516	0	0	0
Maine	100	3	3	3
Maryland	101	0	0	0
Massachusetts	314	0	0	0
Michigan	263	64	46	24
Minnesota	189	0	0	0
Mississippi	298	0	0	0
Missouri	30	0	0	0
Montana	52	0	0	0
Nebraska	88	0	0	0

Dollars in millions

| State | Total state Medicaid payments for physician and surgical services[a] | Non-DSH supplemental payments for physician and surgical services | | Non-DSH supplemental payments as a percentage of state's total for physician and surgical services |
		Total	Federal share	
Nevada	88	4	3	4
New Hampshire	55	0	0	0
New Jersey	63	0	0	0
New Mexico	41	4	4	11
New York	361	0	0	0
North Carolina	944	0	0	0
North Dakota	48	0	0	0
Ohio	317	0	0	0
Oklahoma	402	<1	<1	<1
Oregon	19	0	0	0
Pennsylvania	209	0	0	0
Rhode Island	15	0	0	0
South Carolina	276	46	36	17
South Dakota	60	0	0	0
Tennessee	28	0	0	0
Texas	1,156	45	31	4
Utah	113	17	14	15
Vermont	2	0	0	0
Virginia	197	29	17	15
Washington	193	0	0	0
West Virginia	183	62	50	34
Wisconsin	63	0	0	0
Wyoming	52	0	0	0
Total	**$12,622[b]**	**$522**	**$377**	**4.13**

Source: GAO analysis of CMS-64 expenditure data.

Notes: Amounts represent payments reported during federal fiscal year 2010 and may include adjustments (positive or negative) to payments made during prior fiscal years. CMS provided these data to GAO on December 22, 2011. When a value was greater than 0, but did not round to $1 million or 1 percent, the cell includes the entry "<1."

[a]Total state Medicaid payments for physician and surgical services include both the state and federal share of payments and include all payments made by states to providers, including non-DSH payments as well as regular payments. They do not include expenditures for program administration.

[b]The nationwide total for state Medicaid payments for physician and surgical services includes about $5 million in payments reported by Puerto Rico and the U.S. territories.

**Table 9: Non-DSH Supplemental Payments for Other Practitioners' Services
Reported during Fiscal Year 2010**

Dollars in millions

| State | Total state Medicaid payments for other practitioners' services[a] | Non-DSH supplemental payments for other practitioners' services[b] | | Non-DSH supplemental payments as a percentage of state's total for other practitioners' services |
		Total	Federal share	
Alabama	$40	$0	$0	0
Alaska	17	0	0	0
Arizona	3	0	0	0
Arkansas	17	0	0	0
California	74	0	0	0
Colorado	0	0	0	0
Connecticut	117	0	0	0
Delaware	1	0	0	0
District of Columbia	2	0	0	0
Florida	37	0	0	0
Georgia	31	0	0	0
Hawaii	1	0	0	0
Idaho	42	0	0	0
Illinois	106	0	0	0
Indiana	10	0	0	0
Iowa	53	0	0	0
Kansas	4	<1	<1	10
Kentucky	26	0	0	0
Louisiana	0	0	0	0
Maine	46	1	<1	1
Maryland	10	0	0	0
Massachusetts	29	0	0	0
Michigan	4	0	0	0
Minnesota	148	0	0	0
Mississippi	4	0	0	0
Missouri	12	0	0	0

Dollars in millions

State	Total state Medicaid payments for other practitioners' services[a]	Non-DSH supplemental payments for other practitioners' services[b]		Non-DSH supplemental payments as a percentage of state's total for other practitioners' services
		Total	Federal share	
Montana	14	0	0	0
Nebraska	5	0	0	0
Nevada	10	0	0	0
New Hampshire	15	0	0	0
New Jersey	46	0	0	0
New Mexico	40	0	0	0
New York	232	0	0	0
North Carolina	29	0	0	0
North Dakota	3	0	0	0
Ohio	60	0	0	0
Oklahoma	24	0	0	0
Oregon	25	0	0	0
Pennsylvania	8	0	0	0
Rhode Island	1	0	0	0
South Carolina	27	0	0	0
South Dakota	2	0	0	0
Tennessee	<1	0	0	0
Texas	849	0	0	0
Utah	4	0	0	0
Vermont	<1	0	0	0
Virginia	25	0	0	0
Washington	33	0	0	0
West Virginia	12	0	0	0
Wisconsin	79	0	0	0
Wyoming	7	0	0	0
Total	$2,386[c]	$1	$1	0.04

Source: GAO analysis of CMS-64 expenditure data.

Notes: Amounts represent payments reported during federal fiscal year 2010 and may include adjustments (positive or negative) to payments made during prior fiscal years. CMS provided these data to GAO on December 22, 2011. When a value was greater than 0, but did not round to $1 million or 1 percent, the cell includes the entry "<1."

ªTotal state Medicaid payments for other practitioners' services include both the state and federal share of payments and include all payments made by states to providers, including non-DSH payments as well as regular payments. They do not include expenditures for program administration.

ᵇOther practitioners' services that may be covered by Medicaid vary from state to state and include health-related or remedial care or services, other than physicians' services, provided by licensed practitioners acting within the scope of practice defined under state law. For example, depending on the state, such services could be provided by chiropractors, nurse midwives, nurse practitioners, and others.

ᶜThe nationwide total for state Medicaid payments for other practitioners' services includes less than $1 million in payments reported by Puerto Rico and the U.S. territories.

**Table 10: Non-DSH Supplemental Payments for Intermediate Care Facility Services
Reported during Fiscal Year 2010**

Dollars in millions

| State | Total state Medicaid payments for intermediate care facility services[a] | Non-DSH supplemental payments for intermediate care facility services[b] | | |
		Total	Federal share	Non-DSH supplemental payments as a percentage of state's total for intermediate care facility services
Alabama	$35	$0	$0	0
Alaska	2	0	0	0
Arizona	0	0	0	0
Arkansas	159	0	0	0
California	716	0	0	0
Colorado	28	0	0	0
Connecticut	292	0	0	0
Delaware	31	0	0	0
District of Columbia	69	0	0	0
Florida	334	0	0	0
Georgia	93	0	0	0
Hawaii	9	0	0	0
Idaho	66	0	0	0
Illinois	767	0	0	0
Indiana	309	0	0	0
Iowa	287	0	0	0
Kansas	62	0	0	0
Kentucky	146	0	0	0
Louisiana	472	0	0	0
Maine	59	0	0	0
Maryland	<1	0	0	0
Massachusetts	243	0	0	0
Michigan	0	0	0	0
Minnesota	167	0	0	0
Mississippi	270	0	0	0
Missouri	134	0	0	0
Montana	13	0	0	0

Dollars in millions

State	Total state Medicaid payments for intermediate care facility services[a]	Non-DSH supplemental payments for intermediate care facility services[b]		Non-DSH supplemental payments as a percentage of state's total for intermediate care facility services
		Total	Federal share	
Nebraska	34	0	0	0
Nevada	18	0	0	0
New Hampshire	3	0	0	0
New Jersey	619	0	0	0
New Mexico	25	0	0	0
New York	3,602	0	0	0
North Carolina	499	0	0	0
North Dakota	87	4	3	5
Ohio	826	0	0	0
Oklahoma	124	0	0	0
Oregon	2	0	0	0
Pennsylvania	603	0	0	0
Rhode Island	11	0	0	0
South Carolina	141	0	0	0
South Dakota	25	0	0	0
Tennessee	225	0	0	0
Texas	1,100	0	0	0
Utah	67	0	0	0
Vermont	0	0	0	0
Virginia	271	-5	-3	-2
Washington	141	<0	<0	<0
West Virginia	63	0	0	0
Wisconsin	142	0	0	0
Wyoming	19	0	0	0
Total	**$13,406[c]**	**$-1**	**<$1**	**-0.01**

Source: GAO analysis of CMS-64 expenditure data.

Notes: Amounts represent payments reported during federal fiscal year 2010 and may include adjustments (positive or negative) to payments made during prior fiscal years. CMS provided these data to GAO on December 22, 2011. When a value was greater than 0, but did not round to $1 million or 1 percent, the cell includes the entry "<1." When a value was less than 0, but did not round to ($1) million or (1 percent), the cell includes the entry "<0."

[a]Total state Medicaid payments for intermediate care facility services include both the state and federal share of payments and include all payments made by states to providers, including non-DSH payments as well as regular payments. They do not include expenditures for program administration.

[b]Intermediate care facility services include those provided by facilities serving individuals with intellectual disabilities.

[c]Puerto Rico and the U.S. territories did not report any payments for intermediate care facility services.

Appendix III: Non-DSH Supplemental Medicaid Payments Reported during 2006 and 2010

This appendix provides state-by-state and nationwide information about non-DSH supplemental Medicaid payments reported during 2006 by the states and District of Columbia in comparison to similar payments reported during 2010.[1]

- Table 11 shows the total amount of non-DSH supplemental payments states reported during 2006 and 2010 and the change from 2006 to 2010 in these amounts, both as a dollar amount and as a percentage of the 2006 total.

- Table 12 shows states' reported non-DSH supplemental payments for specific categories of service during 2006 and 2010.

---

[1]Puerto Rico and the U.S. territories that operate Medicaid programs—American Samoa, Guam, the Northern Mariana Islands, and the U.S. Virgin Islands—did not report supplemental Medicaid payments during 2010.

Table 11: Non-DSH Supplemental Payments Reported during Fiscal Years 2006 and 2010

Dollars in millions

State	Total reported non-DSH supplemental payments		Change from 2006 to 2010 in reported non-DSH supplemental payments	
	2006	2010	In dollars	As a percentage of 2006 total
Alabama	$275	$227	$-48	-18
Alaska	30	0	-30	-100
Arizona	0	0	0	0
Arkansas	63	292	229	361
California	1,024	1,786	762	74
Colorado	140	682	542	388
Connecticut	0	0	0	0
Delaware	0	0	0	0
District of Columbia	0	0	0	0
Florida	681	1,485	804	118
Georgia	332	0	-332	-100
Hawaii	18	22	4	21
Idaho	0	0	0	0
Illinois	631	2,659	2,029	322
Indiana	0	178	178	N/A
Iowa	0	0	0	0
Kansas	0	54	54	N/A
Kentucky	0	77	77	N/A
Louisiana	31	0	-31	-100
Maine	0	57	57	N/A
Maryland	0	0	0	0
Massachusetts	0	213	213	N/A
Michigan	13	914	901	6,806
Minnesota	0	0	0	0
Mississippi	175	434	259	149
Missouri	116	0	-116	-100
Montana	33	0	-33	-100
Nebraska	48	0	-48	-100
Nevada	0	39	39	N/A
New Hampshire	19	0	-19	-100

Dollars in millions

State	Total reported non-DSH supplemental payments		Change from 2006 to 2010 in reported non-DSH supplemental payments	
	2006	2010	In dollars	As a percentage of 2006 total
New Jersey	0	0	0	0
New Mexico	49	100	51	103
New York	385	513	129	33
North Carolina	825	218	-608	-74
North Dakota	0	8	8	N/A
Ohio	46	155	109	240
Oklahoma	28	16	-12	-43
Oregon	15	0	-15	-100
Pennsylvania	0	410	410	N/A
Rhode Island	0	0	0	0
South Carolina	335	145	-189	-57
South Dakota	0	0	0	0
Tennessee	127	444	317	251
Texas	818	3,099	2,281	279
Utah	0	17	17	N/A
Vermont	0	<1	<1	N/A
Virginia	0	29	29	N/A
Washington	9	11	1	13
West Virginia	36	137	101	282
Wisconsin	29	0	-29	-100
Wyoming	0	0	0	0
Total	**$6,332**	**$14,420**	**$8,088**	**127.72**

Source: GAO analysis of CMS-64 expenditure data.

Notes: Amounts represent payments reported during federal fiscal years and may include adjustments (positive or negative) to payments made during prior fiscal years. CMS provided the data for fiscal year 2010 to GAO on December 22, 2011. The data for fiscal year 2006 reflect adjustments reported by states through October 5, 2007. When a value was greater than 0, but did not round to $1 million or 1 percent, the cell includes the entry "<1." If a state did not report non-DSH supplemental payments during 2006, but did report such payments during 2010, the percentage change from 2006 could not be computed and is indicated by "N/A."

Table 12: Non-DSH Supplemental Payments States Reported during Fiscal Years 2006 and 2010 by Category of Service

Dollars in millions

State	Inpatient hospital services		Outpatient hospital services		Nursing facility services		Physician and surgical services		Intermediate care facility services[a]		Mental health facility services[b]		Other practitioners' services[c,d]		Other services[b]	
	2006	2010	2006	2010	2006	2010	2006	2010	2006	2010	2006	2010	2006	2010	2006	2010
Alabama	$130	$210	$96	$17	$50	$0	$0	$0	$0	$0	$0	N/A	N/A	$0	$0	N/A
Alaska	30	0	0	0	0	0	0	0	0	0	1	N/A	N/A	0	0	N/A
Arizona	0	0	0	0	0	0	0	0	0	0	0	N/A	N/A	0	0	N/A
Arkansas	63	236	0	46	0	0	0	10	0	0	1	N/A	N/A	0	0	N/A
California	748	1,668	221	96	54	21	0	0	0	0	0	N/A	N/A	0	0	N/A
Colorado	126	417	12	132	2	119	0	15	0	0	0	N/A	N/A	0	<1	N/A
Connecticut	0	0	0	0	0	0	0	0	0	0	0	N/A	N/A	0	0	N/A
Delaware	0	0	0	0	0	0	0	0	0	0	0	N/A	N/A	0	0	N/A
District of Columbia	0	0	0	0	0	0	0	0	0	0	0	N/A	N/A	0	0	N/A
Florida	663	1,334	0	0	18	14	0	137	0	0	0	N/A	N/A	0	0	N/A
Georgia	156	0	65	0	110	0	0	0	0	0	0	N/A	N/A	0	0	N/A
Hawaii	10	18	2	4	6	0	0	0	0	0	0	N/A	N/A	0	0	N/A
Idaho	0	0	0	0	0	0	0	0	0	0	0	N/A	N/A	0	0	N/A
Illinois	474	1,923	156	736	0	0	0	0	0	0	0	N/A	N/A	0	0	N/A
Indiana	0	43	0	0	0	88	0	47	0	0	0	N/A	N/A	0	0	N/A
Iowa	0	0	0	0	0	0	0	0	0	0	0	N/A	N/A	0	0	N/A
Kansas	0	20	0	18	0	0	0	16	0	0	0	N/A	N/A	<1	0	N/A
Kentucky	0	54	0	0	0	<1	0	23	0	0	0	N/A	N/A	0	0	N/A
Louisiana	1	0	13	0	0	0	17	0	0	0	0	N/A	N/A	0	0	N/A
Maine	0	28	0	26	0	0	0	3	0	0	0	N/A	N/A	1	0	N/A
Maryland	0	0	0	0	0	0	0	0	0	0	0	N/A	N/A	0	0	N/A
Massachusetts	0	46	0	167	0	0	0	0	0	0	0	N/A	N/A	0	0	N/A
Michigan	0	428	13	116	0	306	0	64	0	0	0	N/A	N/A	0	0	N/A
Minnesota	0	0	0	0	0	0	0	0	0	0	0	N/A	N/A	0	0	N/A
Mississippi	150	434	20	0	5	0	0	0	0	0	0	N/A	N/A	0	0	N/A
Missouri	70	0	16	0	0	0	5	0	25	0	0	N/A	N/A	0	0	N/A
Montana	27	0	0	0	6	0	0	0	0	0	0	N/A	N/A	0	<1	N/A
Nebraska	0	0	0	0	48	0	0	0	0	0	0	N/A	N/A	0	0	N/A
Nevada	0	35	0	0	0	0	0	4	0	0	0	N/A	N/A	0	0	N/A
New Hampshire	0	0	0	0	19	0	0	0	0	0	0	N/A	N/A	0	0	N/A

Dollars in millions

State	Inpatient hospital services		Outpatient hospital services		Nursing facility services		Physician and surgical services		Intermediate care facility services[a]		Mental health facility services[b]		Other practitioners' services[c,d]		Other services[b]	
	2006	2010	2006	2010	2006	2010	2006	2010	2006	2010	2006	2010	2006	2010	2006	2010
New Jersey	0	0	0	0	0	0	0	0	0	0	0	N/A	N/A	0	0	N/A
New Mexico	0	96	0	0	0	0	0	4	0	0	0	N/A	N/A	0	49	N/A
New York	385	45	0	425	0	44	0	0	0	0	0	N/A	N/A	0	0	N/A
North Carolina	572	218	253	0	0	0	0	0	0	0	0	N/A	N/A	0	0	N/A
North Dakota	0	4	0	0	0	0	0	0	0	4	0	N/A	N/A	0	0	N/A
Ohio	46	155	0	0	0	0	0	0	0	0	0	N/A	N/A	0	0	N/A
Oklahoma	24	16	0	0	0	0	0	<1	0	0	0	N/A	N/A	0	5	N/A
Oregon	10	0	0	0	0	0	4	0	0	0	0	N/A	N/A	0	0	N/A
Pennsylvania	0	0	0	0	0	410	0	0	0	0	0	N/A	N/A	0	0	N/A
Rhode Island	0	0	0	0	0	0	0	0	0	0	0	N/A	N/A	0	0	N/A
South Carolina	205	36	129	24	0	39	0	46	0	0	0	N/A	N/A	0	0	N/A
South Dakota	0	0	0	0	0	0	0	0	0	0	0	N/A	N/A	0	0	N/A
Tennessee	0	444	0	0	127	0	0	0	0	0	0	N/A	N/A	0	0	N/A
Texas	787	3,050	6	4	0	0	25	45	0	0	0	N/A	N/A	0	0	N/A
Utah	0	0	0	0	0	0	0	17	0	0	0	N/A	N/A	0	0	N/A
Vermont	0	0	0	0	0	<1	0	0	0	0	0	N/A	N/A	0	0	N/A
Virginia	0	1	0	0	0	4	0	29	0	-5	0	N/A	N/A	0	0	N/A
Washington	9	<1	0	0	0	11	0	0	0	<0	0	N/A	N/A	0	0	N/A
West Virginia	21	74	0	0	0	0	14	62	0	0	0	N/A	N/A	0	1	N/A
Wisconsin	3	0	<1	0	24	0	0	0	<1	0	<1	N/A	N/A	0	1	N/A
Wyoming	0	0	0	0	0	0	0	0	0	0	0	N/A	N/A	0	0	N/A
Total	$4,711	$11,031	$1,003	$1,811	$469	$1,056	$66	$522	$25	$-1	$2	N/A	N/A	$1	$57	N/A

Source: GAO analysis of CMS-64 expenditure data.

Notes: Amounts represent payments reported during federal fiscal years and may include adjustments (positive or negative) to payments made during prior fiscal years. CMS provided the data for fiscal year 2010 to GAO on December 22, 2011. The data for fiscal year 2006 reflect adjustments reported by states through October 5, 2007. When a value was greater than 0, but did not round to $1 million or 1 percent, the cell includes the entry "<1." When a value was less than 0, but did not round to ($1) million or (1 percent), the cell includes the entry "<0."

[a]Intermediate care facility services include those provided by facilities serving individuals with intellectual disabilities.

[b]The expenditure reporting form used in fiscal year 2010 did not include a way for states to separately report non-DSH supplemental payments for services other than inpatient hospital services, outpatient hospital services, nursing facility services, physician and surgical services, intermediate care facility services, or other practitioners' services. For example, there was no line on which states could report non-DSH supplemental payments for mental health facility services or clinic services. Cells corresponding to categories of service for which no lines were included on the reporting form for 2010—those for mental health facility services and other services—are marked "N/A" (not applicable).

[c]Other practitioners' services that may be covered by Medicaid vary from state to state and include health-related or remedial care or services, other than physicians' services, provided by licensed practitioners acting within the scope of practice defined under state law. For example, depending on the state, such services could be provided by chiropractors, nurse midwives, nurse practitioners, and others.

[d]Although the expenditure reporting form used in fiscal year 2006 included a way for states to separately report non-DSH supplemental payments for other practitioners' services, we designated all non-DSH supplemental payments other than inpatient hospital services, outpatient hospital services, nursing facility services, physician and surgical services, intermediate care facility services, and mental health facility services as payments for other services. Cells corresponding to other practitioners' services for 2006 are marked "N/A" (not applicable).

Appendix IV: Comments from the Department of Health and Human Services

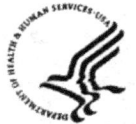

DEPARTMENT OF HEALTH & HUMAN SERVICES

OFFICE OF THE SECRETARY

Assistant Secretary for Legislation
Washington, DC 20201

July 2, 2012

Katherine Iritani
Director, Health Care
U.S. Government Accountability Office
441 G Street NW
Washington, DC 20548

Dear Ms. Iritani:

Thank you for the opportunity to comment on the U.S. Government Accountability Office's (GAO) report entitled: "MEDICAID: States Reported Billions More in Supplemental Payments in Recent Years" (GAO-12-694). Although GAO did not include formal recommendations in this report, it did include an observation that ongoing federal efforts to improve the completeness of reporting of Medicaid supplemental payments are important for effective oversight and to better understand their role in financing Medicaid services. HHS and CMS will continue its ongoing efforts to improve states' reporting of supplemental payments including requiring states to report such payments on their quarterly CMS-64 report.

The Department appreciates the opportunity to review this report prior to publication.

Sincerely,

Jim R. Esquea
Assistant Secretary for Legislation

Appendix V: GAO Contact and Staff Acknowledgments

GAO Contact	Katherine M. Iritani, (202) 512-7114 or iritanik@gao.gov
Staff Acknowledgments	In addition to the contact named above, Tim Bushfield, Assistant Director; Kristen Joan Anderson; Helen Desaulniers; Sandra George; Giselle Hicks; Roseanne Price; and Jessica C. Smith made key contributions to this report.

Related GAO Products

Opportunities to Reduce Potential Duplication in Government Programs, Save Tax Dollars, and Enhance Revenue. GAO-11-318SP. Washington, D.C.: March 1, 2011.

High-Risk Series: An Update. GAO-11-278. Washington, D.C.: February 2011.

Medicaid: Ongoing Federal Oversight of Payments to Offset Uncompensated Hospital Care Costs Is Warranted. GAO-10-69. Washington, D.C.: November 20, 2009.

Medicaid: CMS Needs More Information on the Billions of Dollars Spent on Supplemental Payments. GAO-08-614. Washington, D.C.: May 30, 2008.

Medicaid Financing: Long-standing Concerns about Inappropriate State Arrangements Support Need for Improved Federal Oversight. GAO-08-650T. Washington, D.C.: April 3, 2008.

Medicaid Financing: Long-Standing Concerns about Inappropriate State Arrangements Support Need for Improved Federal Oversight. GAO-08-255T. Washington, D.C.: November 1, 2007.

Medicaid Financing: Federal Oversight Initiative Is Consistent with Medicaid Payment Principles but Needs Greater Transparency. GAO-07-214. Washington, D.C.: March 30, 2007.

Medicaid Financial Management: Steps Taken to Improve Federal Oversight but Other Actions Needed to Sustain Efforts. GAO-06-705. Washington, D.C.: June 22, 2006.

Medicaid Financing: States' Use of Contingency-Fee Consultants to Maximize Federal Reimbursements Highlights Need for Improved Federal Oversight. GAO-05-748. Washington, D.C.: June 28, 2005.

Medicaid: States' Efforts to Maximize Federal Reimbursements Highlight Need for Improved Federal Oversight. GAO-05-836T. Washington, D.C.: June 28, 2005.

Medicaid: Intergovernmental Transfers Have Facilitated State Financing Schemes. GAO-04-574T. Washington, D.C.: March 18, 2004.

Medicaid: Improved Federal Oversight of State Financing Schemes Is Needed. GAO-04-228. Washington, D.C.: February 13, 2004.

Major Management Challenges and Program Risks: Department of Health and Human Services. GAO-03-101. Washington, D.C.: January 2003.

Medicaid: HCFA Reversed Its Position and Approved Additional State Financing Schemes. GAO-02-147. Washington, D.C.: October 30, 2001.

Medicaid: State Financing Schemes Again Drive Up Federal Payments. GAO/T-HEHS-00-193. Washington, D.C.: September 6, 2000.

Medicaid: Disproportionate Share Payments to State Psychiatric Hospitals. GAO/HEHS-98-52. Washington, D.C.: January 23, 1998.

Medicaid: Disproportionate Share Hospital Payments to Institutions for Mental Diseases. GAO/HEHS-97-181R. Washington, D.C.: July 15, 1997.

Medicaid: States Use Illusory Approaches to Shift Program Costs to Federal Government. GAO/HEHS-94-133. Washington, D.C.: August 1, 1994.